CHILD, YOUTH AND FAMILY HEALTH

Strengthening communities

Edited by

Margaret Barnes

Jennifer Rowe

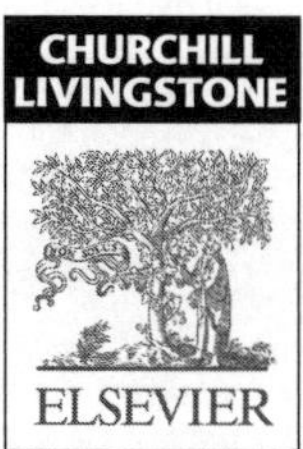

Sydney Edinburgh London New York Philadelphia St Louis Toronto

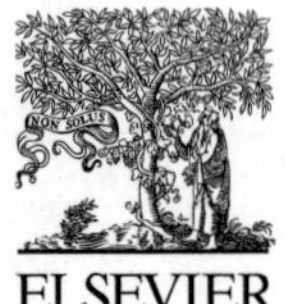

ELSEVIER

Churchill Livingstone
is an imprint of Elsevier

Elsevier Australia
(a division of Reed International Books Australia Pty Ltd)
30–52 Smidmore Street, Marrickville, NSW 2204
ACN 001 002 357

National Library of Australia Cataloguing-in-Publication Data

---

Barnes, Margaret.
Child, youth and family health : strengthening communities.

Bibliography.
Includes index.
ISBN 978-0-7295-3799-5 (pbk.).

1. Child health services - Australia. 2. Medical care - Australia. 3. Family nursing - Australia. I. Rowe, Jennifer. II. Title.

362.70994

Publisher: Debbie Lee
Publishing Services Manager: Helena Klijn
Edited by Ruth Matheson
Proofread by Kay Waters
Internal design and typesetting by Egan-Reid
Cover design by Design Animals
Index by Michael Ferreira
Printed in Australia by Ligare

Printed on paper manufactured from sustainable forests.

Contents

Foreword

It is indeed a pleasure to see a book of this importance written and published.

Child, youth and family health: strengthening communities will be a very valuable resource in schools of nursing and midwifery especially, and to the nursing profession generally.

Given the troubled times in which we live, we need to respect and treasure our children and families, as they are our future.

It is recognised that a culturally competent workforce is required to provide appropriate, relevant care to a broad range of patients/clients from many cultures with the respect that they deserve.

I congratulate the editors and contributors for recognising the need for a text such as this.

Sally Goold OAM
Senior Australian of the Year 2006
Executive Director—Congress of Aboriginal and Torres Strait Islander Nurses

Contributors

Margaret Barnes RN, EM, BEd, MA, PhD
Senior Lecturer, Nursing and Midwifery, University of the Sunshine Coast, Qld

Cheryl Benn RM, RCpN, BSocSc(Hons), MCur, DipNEd, DCur, IBCLC
Associate Professor, Director of Midwifery Programmes, School of Health Sciences, Massey University, NZ

Vicki Bradford RN, GDip Indigenous Health Studies, MA Indigenous Health Studies
Sub-Dean, Indigenous Strategy and Undergraduate, Faculty of Nursing and Midwifery, University of Sydney, NSW

Jon Darvill RN, MN, GCert Higher Ed
Lecturer (adj), Child Youth and Family Nursing, School of Health Sciences, University of Canberra, ACT

Gay Edgecombe RN, RM, CHN, BApplSc, MS, PhD
Clinical Chair, Community Child Health Nursing
Director of International Studies for Nursing and Midwifery, Division of Nursing and Midwifery, School of Health Sciences, RMIT University, Bundoora West Campus, Vic.

Elizabeth Forster RN, BN, MN, GCert Higher Ed, PhD Candidate UQ
Lecturer, School of Nursing, Queensland University of Technology, Qld

Jenny Fraser RN, EM, PhD
Senior Lecturer, School of Nursing, Queensland University of Technology, Qld

Christine Handley RN, BAppSc, MEd, FACMHN, FCNA
Senior Lecturer, School of Nursing and Midwifery, University of Tasmania, Tas.
Child and Adolescent Mental Health Nursing Clinician, CAMHS, DHHS, Tas.

Pamela Henry RN, MN(Hons), PGDip PH
Charge Nurse Manager, Kidz First Homecare Nursing Service, Counties Manukau District Health Board, NZ

Evelyn Hikuroa RN, PGCert Clinical Teaching, PGCert Public Health, MHSc candidate
Senior Lecturer, Department of Nursing and Health Studies, Manukau Institute of Technology, NZ

Sue Kruske RN, RM, BHSc(Hons), GCert Child Health, PhD
Senior Lecturer, Maternal and Child Health, Charles Darwin University, NT

Margaret McAllister RN, RPN, EdD
Associate Professor, School of Health and Sport Sciences, Faculty of Science, Health and Education, University of the Sunshine Coast, Qld

Karen McBride-Henry RN, PhD
Director, Clinical Effectiveness Unit and Senior Lecturer, Graduate School of Nursing and Midwifery, Victoria University of Wellington, NZ

Catherine Maginnis RN, RM, BAppSc(Nurs), MHSc(Nurs), GCert Child Adol Health, MRCNA
Lecturer, School of Nursing and Midwifery, Charles Sturt University, NSW

Judith Murray BA(Hons1), DipEd, BEdSt, PhD
Senior Lecturer, School of Psychology and School of Social Work and Applied Human Sciences, University of Queensland, Qld

Janet Roden RN, CM, BA, MA, PhD, FCN, MRCNA
Lecturer, School of Nursing, University of Western Sydney, NSW

Judith Rorden BSc, BEd, MSc

Jennifer Rowe RN, BA, Dip Ed, GradDipEd (Nurs), MPhil, PhD
Senior Lecturer, School of Nursing and Midwifery, Griffith University, Qld

Linda Shields PhD, MMedSc, BAppSc
Professor of Nursing, Faculty of Health and Social Care, University of Hull, UK
Honorary Professor, Department of Paediatrics and Child Health, University of Queensland, Qld

Lindsay Smith RN, BHlthSc(Nurs), MNS, GradCertUnivLearn&Teach, MRCNA, PhD candidate (Family Health)
Quality of Life & Social Justice Flagship, Australian Catholic University
Lecturer, School of Nursing and Midwifery, University of Tasmania, Tas.

Kay Thomas RN, GCert Paediatric, Child and Youth Health Nursing
Clinical Nurse Consultant, Caring for Kids at Home, Child Youth & Women's Health Program, Community Health, ACT Health, ACT

Reviewers

Barbara Beale RN, RM, MNurs(Hons), BAppScNursing, FRCNA
Lecturer, School of Nursing, University of Western Sydney, NSW

Andrew Gardner RN, RMHN, BN, MMHN, MBA, Dip Medical Hypnosis
Lecturer, School of Nursing and Midwifery, University of South Australia, SA

Michelle Honey RGON, MPhil(Nurs)
Senior Lecturer, School of Nursing, University of Auckland, NZ

Catherine Maginnis RN, RM, BAppSc(Nurs), MHSc(Nurs), GCert Child Adol Health, MRCNA
Lecturer, School of Nursing and Midwifery, Charles Sturt University, NSW

Acknowledgments

Children: they are our past, the present and the future. They are the source of our greatest joy and pleasure, but also our worry and despair. We have been motivated throughout this project by a passion for children and their families—one that has immersed us, professionally and personally, in their lives for many years. So it is a great pleasure to see our efforts come to fruition in this publication.

We have been assisted in this task by a number of people, to whom thanks are due. First, we thank the contributors. At the outset, we knew some of the women and men who have written for this volume, but not all. New relationships have been forged in the process, as we have communicated the needs of the text through telephone, email and, occasionally, in person. All the authors have drawn on their expertise and experience to write and each has contributed to the richness of the text. So we extend our appreciation to Janet, Gay and Karen, Sue, Evelyn and Vicki, Jenny, Judith, Cheryl, Catherine and Linda, Lindsay, Margaret and Christine, Elizabeth and Judith, Jon, Kay and Pamela.

The project has been steered by Debbie Lee from Elsevier, whose commitment, enthusiasm and skill with people has played a pivotal role from proposal to publication. To her and Mae Boadle and the other staff at Elsevier who have played a part, thank you. Good editing is vital, and this role has been fulfilled by Ruth Matheson—thanks and perhaps we shall meet one day. Feedback from anonymous reviewers both of the initial proposal and individual chapters has been an important influence on the final manuscript preparation and we extend our appreciation to them for their thoughtful comments.

Introduction

Margaret Barnes and Jennifer Rowe

Families today are conceptualised as the mortar of society. They do, however, face many challenges, replete with risks to the family as it has been known and risks to family and individual health from a widening range of environmental and lifestyle dynamics. Thus, child, youth and family health services seek to strengthen and support families, prevent illness and manage risks, from both a short-term and long-term perspective.

Healthcare for the child, youth and family in both Australia and New Zealand is publicly funded, with many services delivered through the public sector. At the same time, consumer expectation and interest has motivated a growing private industry—packaged in a range of products, books, information lines, websites and workshops to name a few. The challenge for families is to sift through and interpret the vast array of information and services in a search for helpful support, and to balance the demands of contemporary life and meet their health needs.

The involvement of nurses in the care and health of children, young people and their families has a long history in Australia, New Zealand and other parts of the world. The infant welfare movement in Australia, of which nurses were central service providers, developed in the early twentieth century in response to concerns about high infant mortality, which, together with declining fertility rates, threatened population growth (Mein Smith 1997). Strategies aimed to educate women and to replace traditional childrearing practices with scientific rationality, a newly found concept successful in industry, now applied to the domestic sphere (Selby 1992, Ritson 1997). In New Zealand, Dr Truby King was most influential in the area of maternal and child welfare. A paediatrician, in 1907 he founded the Royal New Zealand Society for the Health of Women and Children, known as the Plunket Society (www.plunket.org.nz). Dr King believed that scientific doctrines regarding nutrition were the only key to reducing the death rate among children and to improving the health of the nation. As with the Australian maternal and child welfare system, his health regime was based on the education and support of mothers and the reliance of 'expert' advice from health professionals, specifically child health nurses.

From these practice beginnings, the scene is set for understanding the development of child health nursing in both Australia and New Zealand today. In both countries, nursing services were developed under the supervision of the medical profession. Nurses were instrumental in implementing programs; however, input into development and planning was limited. This reflects the relationship between medicine and nursing more generally, and it remains a challenge to nursing practice with children, young people and families today.

In the contemporary context, child health services are developed in response to policy and strategy at the national or local level, and are based on priority health areas, with varying levels of input from nurses into this process. The shopfront of practice is diverse, from community and outreach centres and hospitals, to telephone, telemedicine and internet bases. In these settings, nurses are challenged by the question of how to occupy the space between service agendas and family needs—that is, how to maintain a focus on the individual, while also providing targeted, population-based practice (Barnes et al. 2003).

In order to meet these challenges, what are the essentials to practice in this diverse field? Reading this text reveals a broad knowledge and skill base, including:

» knowledge and understanding of health determinants
» knowledge of individual, family and environmental risk and protective factors for health
» appreciation of family and social diversity
» cultural competence
» ability to work with family strengths
» program development and evaluation
» advocacy
» communication
» research appreciation
» clinical competence
» understanding of health literacy, and
» the ability to work with multidisciplinary teams and community groups.

Education for child and youth health nursing practice varies across Australia and New Zealand, with most programs being conducted at the postgraduate level. Education for community practice considers the role of the nurse as an autonomous professional working within a multidisciplinary team. It is advanced and specialised.

In Queensland, Australia, for example, the School Based Youth Health Program employs nurses to provide individual consultation, health promotion and support to high school students. Issues facing young people are reflected in case management, with nurses frequently supporting young people with mental health problems, drug and alcohol issues, or sexual health concerns. This practice is often within an environment where resources are scarce and referral delayed by lack of services or remote geography. This is just one example. Many more are provided in this text—in acute settings and for children with chronic disease across the home–hospital interface, as well as with groups of well infants and children and their families.

In writing this text, we have attempted to provide a foundation for working with the child, young person and the family across a range of health contexts and life stages. In providing this forum, we hope to highlight the valuable nursing work that occurs with these client groups, the range of settings and the level of skill required. A strengths approach is adopted. This is an attempt to reframe the construction of nursing practice in child, youth and family health from a bureaucratic model to a collaborative and partnership model, centred on working with families where they are and with the strengths they have. The text adopts a critical lens, so as to not only describe practice but also to highlight challenges and issues for readers to consider.

The book is organised in two parts. Part A provides a broad-brush approach to issues facing the health and wellbeing of children and young people. The place of family in society, culture and healthcare is discussed in Chapter 1. As nurses need to meet the challenge of increasing their leadership through engagement in policy, service and program initiatives, the keys for effectiveness are set out in Chapter 2. Developing programs with the health service, in response to community need, is discussed.

In Chapter 3, there is an emphasis on the particular needs of Indigenous peoples, including a reflection on the social and political circumstance that has led to what continues to be poorer health and wellbeing than the rest of the population in both Australia and New Zealand. Ethical and legal dimensions of practice are complex and essential. The reader is challenged in Chapter 4 to consider these dimensions within the overarching practice imperative of advocacy. Working with infants, young children and young people and their families requires advanced communication skills. These are discussed in Chapter 5.

Part B focuses more closely on the practice context and provides a wide range of situations in which nurses and midwives practise directly or indirectly to improve health outcomes. Chapters 6 and 7 focus upon the developing family, particularly women and parents during pregnancy and the first year of a child's life, as supportive services are critical to promoting healthy families. Chapter 8 focuses on toddlers and young children. The importance of family as guides and carers both in health and illness are highlighted in the discussion. The interface of home, school and healthcare to promote wellbeing in young children is explored.

Youth health has received a recent and timely refocusing of attention and services. Recognition of the social and health issues facing young people has led to the development of national policy and strategic directions. Young people face a number of physical, developmental, psychological or behavioural challenges, and the problems of alcohol and drug use and abuse, sexual behaviour, mental health problems, delinquency and violence mean that young people are increasingly vulnerable. These issues and the challenges for nurses working with young people are discussed in Chapters 9 and 10.

Two important and discrete areas of practice form the basis of Chapters 11 and 12. In Chapter 11, grief and loss are examined and the reader is given the opportunity to understand grief and loss from the position of children of different ages, and family members. Finally, but not least, in Chapter 12, chronic illness in childhood is examined. Through two very different scenarios, the reader is taken into the world of the family who has a child with an ongoing health problem. The complexities of service and practice are discussed showing the multiple, collaborative and partnership basis of effective healthcare.

References

Barnes M, Courtney M, Pratt J, Walsh A 2003 Contemporary child health nursing practice: services provided and challenges faced in metropolitan and outer Brisbane areas. *Collegian* 10(4):14–19.

Mein Smith P 1997 *Mothers and King baby: infant survival and welfare in an imperial world: Australia 1880–1950*. Macmillan, London.

Ritson R 1997 The birth of the clinic. *Transition* 54(55):42–53.

Selby W 1992 Motherhood in Labor's Queensland 1915–1957. Unpublished PhD thesis. Griffith University, Nathan, Queensland.

Part A

Issues and challenges in child, youth and family health

Chapter 1

Locating the child, young person and family in contemporary healthcare

Margaret Barnes, Jennifer Rowe and Janet Roden[1]

Learning outcomes

Reading this chapter will help you to:

- » understand the nature of the contemporary family
- » appreciate family diversity
- » locate the family within contemporary society
- » understand the changing nature of the family
- » discuss health determinants as they relate to children and young people
- » understand the influence of social gradient on child health and the implications for health later in life
- » identify current child and youth health priorities, and
- » demonstrate an understanding of the importance of family assessment.

Introduction

Working with children and young people is both rewarding and challenging. Nurses and midwives caring for this client group do so, most commonly, within the context of the family. It is important therefore to understand the nature and shape of the family as a mediator and facilitator for children and young people,

1 The authors would like to acknowledge the contribution to this chapter from Mr Lindsay Smith for the material on family assessment (pp 11–14).

their health and wellbeing. This chapter, therefore, situates the child, young person and family in contemporary New Zealand and Australian society and examines the underpinnings of children and young people's health and healthcare in these countries.

As background to this, an overview of how the family as it is both constructed and how it functions today is provided. Societal approaches to capturing health priorities and developing policy to strengthen individual and family health is outlined. A strengths framework is adopted in order to set the scene for understanding and assessing children's health needs. This framework places emphasis on working with families and individuals to achieve optimal health outcomes for children and young people.

Contemporary impressions of the family and community

Family life has changed over recent decades in both Australia and New Zealand with a rise in divorce, increasing workforce participation by both parents, and single parenting. Such changes have brought into question the quality of family life, especially for children. However, historical analysis tends to point to the importance of a longer term view of family development (Featherstone 2004). The nature and pattern of family life have changed over time and have probably done so for centuries.

Early in the twenty-first century the focus, however, tends to be nostalgic for the 1950s, an era that seems to be considered the benchmark for ideal family life. An understanding and critique of trends in family life are therefore important, as they influence and shape the way health professionals may view family functioning and child health and, more broadly, how governments prioritise social and health policy and service provision.

Any discussion of the family needs to be prefaced with contemporary working definitions. There are a number of definitions of family that can inform thinking about family within the context of child, youth and family health. For example, for the purpose of census data collection, the ABS (Australian Bureau of Statistics 2002) defines family as:

> 'Two or more persons, one of whom is aged 15 years and over, who are related by blood, marriage (registered or de facto), adoption, step or fostering: and who are usually resident in the same household.'

In New Zealand, and again in the context of social statistics, one definition suggests that the family 'consists of a couple, with or without children, or one parent with children, usually living together in a household. Couples can be same sex or opposite-sex' (Statistics New Zealand 2004 p. 1). It is clear that, in these constructions, the family is about household, and the child and young person are optional rather than integral, and it is certainly far from the idealised 1950s family.

Discussion about the family within the nursing context, however, requires a broad definition. For example, Wright and Leahey suggest that 'the family is who they say they are' (2005 p. 60). While the definitions of family vary, it is important to understand the social, cultural and political factors that might shape the way family is considered. There may be an ideal image of a family embedded in our thinking about families, but the reality is that the nature and shape of families is dynamic and the result of decades, and centuries, of social change. Family diversity then is a response to changing times.

Gilding (2001) observes that there have been a number of distinct eras in family structure in postcolonial Australia. The first was the era of federation, over a century ago, when families were enmeshed in wider relationships. They may have produced a variety of goods and services in the home and opened their home to guests and extended family. Middle class households employed servants (domestic service being the main source of employment for women). For the working class family, households were commonly overcrowded, experiencing difficult economic circumstances.

This was a time of declining birthrate, one of the responses to which was the infant welfare movement. The declining birthrate was blamed on the 'selfishness' of women who would prefer the luxuries of life over rearing children (Royal Commission 1904 p. 17, cited in Gilding 2001). This decline was the cause of a moral panic about the population and about women's role in the family and society. In addition, the declining birthrate was a concern in both countries as each sought to develop a labour force. The effect was increased surveillance of mothering and an increasing separation of the domestic and private from the commercial and public space.

The postwar decades of the 1950s and 1960s saw the predominance of the nuclear family and the dominance of western values, despite the increasing ethnic diversity in each country. Women became 'housewives' as fewer servants were employed and households were more likely to be a single family, and the growth of the welfare state meant that financial support was more readily available (Gilding 2001). This era promoted marriage and the family and is often reflected upon as the time of the 'traditional' family (Gilding 2001).

In the following decades there was significant change occurring to the family. During the 1970s and 1980s there was increasing diversity, women increasingly entered the workforce, children stayed at home and at school longer, and it was the age of sexual liberation. It was a time when there were fewer marriages, more de facto relationships, more divorce and fewer children (Gilding 2002). There was also increasing diversity in migrant families and therefore ethnicity (Poole 2005). For some, the family had undergone irreparable change.

Over a century of change, diversity and panic about the family, and more recent fears from politicians and the media, have led to fear that the family is in decline. In 2003, in Australia, however, 87% of the population lived in family households (Australian Bureau of Statistics 2004). The family is not in decline as such, but the characteristics of the family have changed. For example, the family of the twenty-first century is characterised by the activities and products of a technological age (Gilding 2002).

The shape of the contemporary twenty-first century family is expected to change further, with concerns of population decline, as the number of couple-only families is predicted to increase and the number of couple families with children is predicted to decline over the next decade (Australian Bureau of Statistics 2004). During this time it is predicted, also, that one-parent families will remain stable, a picture that tends to contrast with expectations and rhetoric that the one-parent family is more common than couple families.

The family characteristics survey conducted in Australia in 2003 demonstrates the diversity of family types within Australia. Families were identified as comprising couples with or without children, lone parents with children or families comprising related adults (Australian Bureau of Statistics 2004). At the time of the survey, 60% of families were families with children, with 79% of the children classed as dependent children. Of families with at least one child aged 0–17 years, 71% were intact couple families, 22% were one-parent families, 4% step-families and 3% blended families (Australian Bureau of Statistics 2004). Important to note is that 23% of children in the 0–17 age group were living in circumstances were a natural parent was living elsewhere (i.e. as a result of separation). A growing family group is that of grandparent families, with over 22,000 identifying as such in 2003. In this group, the younger partner was younger than 55 years in 39% of families, with the majority being over 55 years.

New Zealand projections (Statistics New Zealand 2004) estimate that trends in family types up to 2021 will see a growth in couples without children and one-parent families (up to approximately 26%) and a decrease in two-parent families. In 2001, 84% of two-parent families and 77% of one-parent families had dependent children. The 2006 New Zealand census data (Statistics New Zealand 2006) suggest that 42% of families are couples with children and 39.9% are couples without children, while 18.1% are one-parent families.

To explore your understanding of 'family', consider the critical questions and reflections in Box 1.1.

Box 1.1 Critical questions and reflections: the 'family'

1. How do you imagine the 'family' within your own social and cultural context?
2. What and who has influenced your family picture?
3. To what extent does understanding of the family contribute to nursing practice?

Social mapping

Try to map your family and relationships to informal and formal community (e.g. schools, health and human services, retail and professional services) and try to imagine and indicate the mechanisms for getting and giving support to members of your social map.

There are many ways to create social, mind or concept maps. It is important to include all the important elements, and to show the relationships among and relative position of each element. A number of websites can give you ideas about how to create them. Enter the search term 'social mapping' in Google to find some.

It is important to understand the evolving and dynamic nature of family and household structures, which change over time, as do fertility patterns, social attitudes and longevity (de Vaus 2004). What we consider the concept of 'family' now will change and may be different from our own perception of what family structure should be. Important for health professionals is an awareness of the diverse types of family and household structures, to be aware of the vulnerabilities and strengths of particular families and to focus on the strengths of that family and household within the context of child health and parenting.

Valuing family diversity

Discussion in this chapter has emphasised the diverse nature of the contemporary family. When discussing family diversity, terms that describe family type or structure (e.g. two-parent families and step-families) often come to mind. However, this approach has the potential to label or stereotype that family in terms of functioning and health. An alternative way to view diversity is explored by Rapoport and Rapoport (1982, in Saggers & Simms 2005) who describe five types of family diversity:

1. Organisational diversity includes the changing patterns of work within and outside the home, and changing marital trends, as described above.
2. Cultural diversity includes Indigenous families, migrant families and refugee families.
3. Social class diversity refers to the material resources of the family, the socialisation and education of children, and relationships between members.
4. Life cycle diversity reflects the life cycle stage within families and includes members from different historical periods.
5. Family lifecourse diversity refers to the different stages a family may be going through (e.g. the family with a new baby, older children or when children leave home).

The sources of diversity describe the way in which families differ as they develop and change over time. Diversity enriches families and society and is valued as contributing to the fabric of the community. Understanding family diversity means understanding the family's background, history and social connections. To explore these concepts further, consider the critical questions and reflections in Box 1.2.

Box 1.2 Critical questions and reflections: family diversity

Consider the types of family diversity as described by Rapoport and Rapoport (1982, in Saggers & Simms 2005). Examine the way in which these sources of diversity may influence the way a family develops, and the way members of the family might respond to health and illness situations.

Risk and protection: individual, family and community factors

Appreciating family diversity leads to an understanding of how families are shaped and how they function within the community—factors that may influence a child's health and wellbeing. These are described as risk and protective factors and relate not only to family factors but also to individual and community ones. Examine the information in Table 1.1. Here you can see the interplay of a diverse range of factors in the family and also the community beyond the family as they potentially influence a child's health and wellbeing. You can see also the multiple, complex and interdependent nature of these factors.

Table 1.1 Risk and protective factors for child development, health and wellbeing in early childhood

Risk factors	Category	Protective factors
Young maternal age Low birthweight Preterm Birth injury/trauma Congenital anomalies Chromosomal abnormalities	Perinatal maternal health Fetal growth Birth	Good maternal perinatal health Antenatal care and screening Uncomplicated vaginal birth
Child illness Maternal illness Poor attachment Prone sleeping Smoke-filled environment Poor nutrition Discontinuity in primary caregivers Maternal depression	Early parenting Infant health	Breastfeeding exclusively to 6 months Good maternal health and nutrition Secure attachment Continuity in and nurturing primary caregivers Immunisation
Low social gradient Low parent education levels Family violence Unstable family Stress and ineffective coping Single parent family Death of family member Family isolation	Family factors	Stable home/family Middle to higher social gradient Parent education Effective coping strategies for stressors Adequate support networks Spacing of any siblings >2 years
Pollution War/natural disaster Lack of health and social service access Inadequate housing, sanitation and water supply	Community factors	Good community cultural identity Community health and social infrastructure Good balance of built and natural community environment

Source: Developed from Blum et al. (2002), National Health and Medical Research Council (NHMRC) and Child and Youth Health Intergovernmental Partnership (CHIP) (2002), Prevatt (2003) and Spencer (2000).

Health determinants and health policy related to children and young people

There is an increasing recognition of the importance of providing services for children and families, with prevention, support and early intervention becoming policy lynchpins (Child and Youth Health Intergovernmental Partnership 2005, Ministry of Health New Zealand 1998). The New Zealand Well Child Tamariki Ora Framework, for instance, sets out the following agenda:

> '. . . the primary objective . . . is to support families/whānau to maximise their child's developmental potential and health status from birth to five years to establish a strong foundation for ongoing healthy development' (Ministry of Health New Zealand 2006).

This approach has coincided with international recognition that children's health is not just a matter of providing services responsive to illness, but that the experiences of early childhood can have a 'profound lifelong impact on a child's health, well-being and competence' (Hertzman 2002 p. 1).

Relationship of social gradient and child health

Increasingly, the relationship between social gradient and the health of children is being recognised, with recognition that social factors have a profound impact on child health (Spencer 2000). Poorer children are at an increased risk of mortality and morbidity in both developed and developing countries, and such mortality and morbidity includes what is considered the 'new' morbidities (Spencer 2000). Graham and Power (2004 p. 671) suggest that 'socio-economic inequalities in health persist even in rich societies where life expectancy is high'. (The term 'new' morbidities refers to the range of factors that influence child health and reflect social and lifestyle factors. They differ from the 'old' causes of illness and death, such as malnutrition and infection, and include accident and injury and behavioural problems.)

Disadvantage influences health in childhood, but, importantly, such disadvantage early in life is increasingly being linked with later adult health. As Graham and Power (2004 p. 673) describe it, 'childhood origins shape adult destinations' and underlying these generational continuities are the educational and social trajectories along which children steer their way to adulthood. The lifecourse framework described by Graham and Power (2004) for considering childhood disadvantage and later adult health includes the important factors of social identity, cognition and education, health behaviour and physical and emotional health.

The evidence suggests that the link between childhood disadvantage and poor adult health can be described as having four elements and is a dynamic and interactive process. The four elements are poor childhood circumstances, a set of interlocking child-to-adult pathways, poor adult circumstances and poor adult health (Graham & Power 2004).

Health priorities

Given these complex and interdependent principles influencing the health of children, it is clear that improving child health is a priority in the goal of improving health overall. However, the greatest challenge is addressing the inequalities and disadvantage that influence child health. If such disadvantage was addressed, the overall health of a society would be positively impacted. With ample evidence pointing to the importance of child health, beginning with healthy pregnancy and maternal health, national policy and strategy is developed to provide a framework for the development of services, infrastructure support and intersectoral collaboration.

The Australian context

In Australia, the aforementioned aspirations for children's health are captured in the *National public health strategic framework for children 2005–2008* (National Public Health Partnership 2005). This framework:

- » seeks to strengthen the capacity of the health sector and the wider community to respond to a range of public health issues identified in national strategies for children aged 0–12 years, including maternal health and wellbeing during the antenatal period
- » is based on health promotion and illness prevention, including early intervention approaches
- » emphasises opportunities to address health inequalities
- » provides a response framework for emerging child public health issues
- » serves to link strategic effort across the various settings and systems involved in the health and wellbeing of children
- » focuses on strengthening the capacity of systems to support communities, families, parents and professionals to support the health of children, and
- » provides a focus on the role of health services.

Development of such national policy is based on multidisciplinary research, an example of which is provided in Box 1.3. Complete the activity to gain an understanding of the ongoing research in this area.

Box 1.3 Research highlight: multidisciplinary health research

Go to the Telethon Institute for Child Health Research at www.ichr.uwa.edu.au/. Examine the site. The Institute is led by Professor Fiona Stanley. Set up in 1990, it is a good example of an influential and multidisciplinary approach to epidemiological clinical and intervention research that promotes children's health and wellbeing in areas of health priorities.

The New Zealand context

The *New Zealand child health strategy* was a 10-year plan launched in 1998. The contributing documents, the *Child health programme review* and *Our children's health* (Ministry of Health New Zealand 1998), were also released at that time. The strategy was developed to reflect the child health community's views about what was needed to improve health outcomes for children/tamariki and their families and whanau in New Zealand.

The future directions outlined in the strategy included:

- » a greater focus on health promotion, prevention and early intervention
- » better coordination
- » the development of a national child health information strategy
- » child health workforce development
- » improvements in child health evaluation and research, and
- » leadership in child health.

At the time of writing, this policy is in review. Limited information about likely policy and service direction is available via the Well Child homepage at www.moh.govt.nz/wellchild.

Family assessment: working with children, young people and families

The application of broad policy frameworks in practice through program development and service delivery is described throughout the chapters in this text. Nurses and midwives are integral to these services and programs. To practise effectively, nurses need to be equipped with a range of competencies and attributes described in the Introduction. Among these competencies is the ability to undertake a comprehensive family assessment and to recognise the interplay of family, community and environment on children's health.

Assessing families is an important aspect of working with children and young people, as it is within the context of the family that care is commonly provided. In the following section, the concept of family assessment is discussed, and a framework and process provided. However, it is important to be aware also of situations when care for children and young people is provided outside the family. A specific example is that of homeless youth, who may be living in circumstances outside the family and have particular health, social and financial concerns.

Neabel et al. (2000) justify the importance of nurses and midwives conducting comprehensive family assessments so that they better understand the family's experience of health or an illness event. Undertaking a thorough family assessment enables the development of an understanding of the family unit, what the health or illness event means to the family members, and identifies what they need. A range of family assessment tools is available, each with different aims and scope. It is important to evaluate such tools as fit for purpose and to critique their ability to achieve their stated aims.

Until recently, family assessment has been dominated by what Feeley and Gottlieb (2000) describe as a deficit-oriented, disorder-oriented or problem-oriented approaches to clinical practice in the helping professions, in that the focus has been on what is missing, what is wrong or abnormal. An alternative approach considers what the family knows and what they can do. This strengths-based approach focuses on the client or family competencies, resources and capacities, and actively seeks to identify strengths within individuals and families (Feeley & Gottlieb 2000). As well, this approach leads to the development of clinician and client relationships based on partnership. (The important role of partnership in child, youth and family work is expanded across the chapters in the text.)

Valuing and assessing family strengths in nursing practice

The strengths-based perspective is a recent development in applied health research and clinical practice. Strengths-based research identifies what individuals, families and communities are doing well and what they can do to enhance resilience. All families have strengths that nurses can draw on through primary healthcare and health promotion activities. There is a growing trend in nursing to understand clinical practice from a family-strengths framework (DeFrain 1999). The strengths framework is a positive approach looking at how families and individuals succeed and promote resilience.

> 'A strengths approach has many benefits to nurses . . . it is essential therefore that nurses engage in the discourses about family-focused approaches and consider the potential benefits of using a strengths approach to understanding resilience and build health capacity in families' (Darbyshire & Jackson 2005 p. 211).

Consequently, it is now time for nurses working with children and families to adopt aspects of the strengths perspective into their clinical practice.

At the core of the strengths framework is the concept that families function best through operational strengths that afford benefits. The best definition is that strengths are:

> '. . . the set of relationships and processes that support and protect families and family members, especially during times of adversity and change. Family strengths help to maintain family cohesion while also supporting the development and wellbeing of individual family members' (Moore et al. 2002 p. 3).

Fundamental principles of the strengths perspective are:

- Each individual, all families and every community have strengths.
- These strengths develop over time.
- Strengths can be encouraged.
- Strengths are vital for optimising outcomes through challenging times, stressful periods and illness (Olson & DeFrain 2006).

The Australian Family Strengths Research Project (Geggie et al. 2000), the first Australian research to identify the language Australians use when talking about their strengths, identified eight qualities of strong Australian families, seven of which were family strengths. The eighth quality, resilience, captures the family's ability to withstand and rebound from crisis and adversity. The eight qualities are:

- communication
- togetherness
- sharing activities
- affection
- support
- acceptance
- commitment, and
- resilience.

Not all families demonstrate similar strengths and how each family demonstrates their strengths may differ from one family to another. Uniting families is a positive emotional connectedness towards one another, causing people in strong families to sacrifice for each other's wellbeing (Olson & DeFrain 2006). Connectedness relates to how attached the individual feels towards the others in the family, as well as how attached the individual feels the other family members are to them.

The Australian Family Strengths Nursing Assessment Guide

Helping families identify and develop their strengths can instigate change in family functioning and increase family resilience (Patterson 2002). Nurses can easily recognise strengths while listening to families tell their story. Nurses can also observe strengths in the family's behaviour in response to the healthcare needs and challenges facing them. Using the language that Australian families use, the Australian Family Strengths Nursing Assessment Guide (Table 1.2) can be used to initiate conversations with any family member that look for, support and encourage family strengths. The questions are asked as if concerning the family as a whole. For example, 'Tell me about when you talk openly with each other' refers to when the members of the family talk openly together. However, these questions can be adapted to suit particular family and individual circumstances.

Table 1.2 Australian Family Strengths Nursing Assessment Guide
Togetherness • In your family, what shared beliefs really matter to you? • Do you share beliefs that really matter together that you would like to follow during this admission/time of healthcare? • What are some of the things that cause you to celebrate together? • Tell me about some of your family's shared memories.
Sharing activities • When does the family spend time together? • What is it you like about when you plan activities together? • How often would you play together as a family? • Tell me about when you have good times together in your family.
Affection • In your family, when is it most easy to tell others how you feel about them? • How best do you show your love for each other? • In what ways do you demonstrate consideration for each other? • How would others know you care about each other? • If I were to ask your best friend about how you care about each other, what would they say? • What sort of things do you do for each other?
Support • Tell me of times when you as a family 'share the load'. • How would an observer seeing your family know that you help each other? • Can you think of ways you look out for each other? • What does it mean in your family to be 'there for each other'? • In what ways do you encourage others to try new things?
Communication • When do you listen to each other? • Tell me about when you talk openly with each other. • Tell me about some of the times when you laugh together. *cont.*

Table 1.2 Australian Family Strengths Nursing Assessment Guide—*cont.*
Acceptance • In what ways do you accept your individual differences? • When are you most likely to give each other space? • How do you show the members of your family that you respect each other's point of view? • What does forgiveness of each other look like in your family? • What different responsibilities does each of you have?
Commitment • When do you feel safe and secure with each other? • How would others know that you trust each other? • List some of the things your family does for your community. • What rules do you have in your family and how should these be followed during this admission?
Resilience • In what ways has this admission changed your plans? • What helps keep each other hopeful? • Can you tell me about when your family pulled together in a crisis? • When you have a problem, what helps you discuss your problems? • What do other people say they admire in your family?

Source: These questions were developed by Smith (2007) based on Geggie et al. (2000), with permission from *Our scrapbook of strengths* (Family Action Centre & St Luke's Innovative Resources 2003), using the language that Australian families use when talking about their own family.

The Australian Family Strengths Nursing Assessment Guide contains questions that can be asked of a child, young person or their family that assist in generating conversations. Through identifying the strengths that a family use, nurses may highlight for the first time that each family member offers something of value to each other, thus increasing the family's sense of purpose and unity. Recognising and encouraging family strengths helps demonstrate an understanding of the whole family's needs and hopes. Walking with the family in this way creates a connectedness that is unique to the relationship. Attempt the activity in Box 1.4 to apply the principles described to practice, and see Chapter 9 for further application of the family strengths perspective with the young person.

Box 1.4 Practice highlight: assessing family strengths
Utilising the Australian Family Strengths Nursing Assessment Guide, engage in a conversation with a family as a group about their strengths and how their family functions across the eight qualities. Explore what goals the family are currently striving towards. Remember, not every strength needs to be explored with every family.

Solution-focused nursing: an example of a strengths-based approach

A complementary approach and a recent development in the attitude and practice of nursing is solution-focused nursing (SFN) (McAllister 2007). A solution-focused approach to interactions with children, young people and their families has capacity building and support as its core (Rowe & Barnes 2007). A solution-focused framework emphasises strengths and goal setting, and focuses on what is of value to the child and family. SFN practice concerns itself with a shift in approach among clinicians to become solution-searchers rather than problem-finders (McAllister 2007). The six principles of SFN are (McAllister 2007):

1. The person rather than the problem is at the centre of inquiry.
2. Look for and work with strengths and resources.
3. Resilience is as important as vulnerability.
4. There is a move from illness-care to adaptation and recovery.
5. The goal is to create change at three levels: the client, nursing and society.
6. The way of being with clients is proactive, rather than reactive.

SFN provides a framework for working with family strengths. An example of the way in which nurses might approach family assessment and care from this perspective is provided in Box 1.5.

Box 1.5 Practice highlight: summary for a solution-focused approach to nursing with families and parents in transition

- First, assess the situation. Is the immediate issue indicative of a specific need for new knowledge, affirmation or caregiving help?
- Put aside your assumptions of what is a priority, or a correct way to go about parenting.
- Be curious and interested in the parents, children, infants and other family members.
- Find out what is going well for the parent. How does the parent judge success?
- Encourage storytelling (e.g. small stories about what the parent is doing, how the parent feels). Ask for illustrations of things that are going well.
- Many beliefs are embedded in people's stories, and stories provide rich material for questioning and opportunities for reinterpreting and seeking solutions.
- Assess the resources the parent may be able to draw on. Help them to work out how to draw on those resources and identify others that may be available and potentially useful.
- Use positive feedback and compliments that are affirming
- Consider closely whether issues raised by parents about caregiving/nurturing are about their identity as parents or about other aspects of their lifestyle.
- Help the parent to be forward looking to reinterpret the present with the future in mind, even when this may be the next day or the next week.
- Ask questions that signpost or construct signposts of vision and success.
- The focus is on realistic goals and small steps, using things that will work for the person.
- Make plans with the person.
- Assess progress—adaptation, motivation, tasks achieved, resources working.

Source: Rowe and Barnes (2007), in M McAllister (ed.), *Solution focused nursing. Rethinking practice.* Palgrave, Houndmills, UK, pp. 49–62.

Conclusion

In this chapter, we have outlined the way in which the family is perceived today. In doing this, contemporary definitions of family are provided, and the dynamic and changing nature of the family discussed. Importantly, discussion of child health priorities is underpinned by an understanding of the influence of social gradient on child health as well as health in later life. Understanding these concepts is essential to practice where policy and programs are driven by epidemiological and demographic data.

Working with children, young people and families requires an understanding of the interplay between social, community and family influences, biology and the environment, as risk or protective factors for health and wellbeing. Understanding risk and protective factors informs approaches to program development, service delivery and individual interactions, and can be applied in strengths-based family assessment and nursing intervention programs.

Key points

» The contemporary family is changing and dynamic.
» Your view of what constitutes 'family' may be different from that of others.
» There is significant social and cultural diversity in families.
» A number of interdependent individual, family and community factors serve risk and protective functions for the developing child's health and wellbeing.
» Social gradient influences child health.
» Childhood disadvantage influences adult health.
» Health priorities and targets are determined at international, national and local levels.
» Strengths-based family assessment approaches provide skills for nurses to work in partnership with families to shape family function and increase resilience.
» Solution-focused nursing approaches work with family strengths to help families meet their healthcare needs.

Useful resources

Australian Bureau of Statistics: www.abs.gov.au.
Australian Institute of Family Studies: www.aifs.gov.au.
New Zealand Government. *New Zealand families today*. Available at www.msd.govt.nz/work-areas/families-whanau/nz-families-today.html.

References

Australian Bureau of Statistics (ABS) 2002 *Census of population and housing. Selected social and housing characteristics, Australia*. Cat. No. 215.0. ABS, Canberra.
Australian Bureau of Statistics (ABS) 2004 *Family characteristics, Australia*. Available at www.abs.gov.au/Austats/abs.nsf/.

Blum RW, McNeely C, Nonnemaker J 2002 Vulnerability, risk and protection. *Journal of Adolescent Health* 31S:28–39.

Child and Youth Health Intergovernmental Partnership (CHIP) 2005 *The strategic framework, healthy children—strengthening promotion and prevention across Australia. National Public Health Strategic Framework for Children 2005–2008.* Available at www.nphp.gov.au/workprog/chip/documents/.

Darbyshire P, Jackson D 2005 Using a strengths approach to understand resilience and build health capacity in families. *Contemporary Nurse* 18(1–2):211–12.

DeFrain J 1999 Strong families around the world. *Family Matters* 53:8.

de Vaus D 2004 *Diversity and change in Australian families. Statistical profiles.* Australian Institute of Family Studies, Melbourne.

Family Action Centre and St Luke's Innovative Resources 2003 *Our scrapbook of strengths.* Pyrenees Press, Maryborough.

Featherstone B 2004 *Family life and family support. A feminist analysis.* Palgrave, Houndmills, UK.

Feeley N, Gottlieb L 2000 Nursing approaches for working with family strengths and resources. *Journal of Family Nursing* 6(1):9–24.

Geggie J, DeFrain J, Hitchcock S, Silberberg S 2000 *The family strengths research report.* Family Action Centre, University of Newcastle.

Gilding M 2001 Changing families in Australia 1901–2001. *Family Matters* 60:6–11.

Gilding M 2002 Families of the new millennium. Designer babies, cyber sex and virtual communities. *Family Matters* 62:4–10.

Graham H, Power C 2004 Childhood disadvantage and health inequalities: a framework for policy based on lifecourse research. *Child: Care, Health and Development* 30(6):671–8.

Hertzman C 2002 *An early child development strategy for Australia. Lessons from Canada,* Issue Paper 1, Commission for Children and Young People, Queensland Government.

McAllister M 2007 An introduction to solution-focused nursing. In M McAllister (ed.), *Solution focused nursing. Rethinking practice.* Palgrave, Houndmills, UK, pp. 49–62.

Ministry of Health New Zealand (MOH NZ) 1998 *New Zealand child health strategy.* MOH NZ, Wellington.

Ministry of Health New Zealand (MOH NZ) 2006 *New Zealand child health strategy,* MOH NZ, Wellington. Available at www.moh.govt.nz/childhealth.

Moore K, Chalk R, Scarpa J, Vandivere S 2002 *Preliminary research on family strengths: A Kids Count working paper.* Annie E Casey Foundation, Maryland.

National Health and Medical Research Council (NHMRC), Child and Youth Health Intergovernmental Partnership (CHIP) 2002 *Child health screening and surveillance: a critical review: supplementary document-context and next steps,* NHMRC, Canberra.

National Public Health Partnership 2005 *Healthy children—strengthening promotion and prevention across Australia. National public health strategic framework for children 2005–2008.* Available at www.dhs.vic.gov.au/nphp/workprog/chip/cyhactionplanbg.htm.

Neabel B, Fothergill-Bourbonnais F, Dunning J 2000 Family assessment tools: a review of the literature from 1978–1997. *Heart and Lung: The Journal of Acute and Critical Care* 29(3):19–209.

Olson D, DeFrain J 2006 *Marriage and the family: intimacy, diversity and strengths*, 5th edn. McGraw-Hill, New York.

Patterson J 2002 Understanding family resilience. *Journal of Clinical Psychology* 58(3):233–46.

Poole M 2005 Changing families, changing times. In M Poole (ed.), *Family: changing families and changing times*. Allen & Unwin, Sydney, pp. 1–19.

Prevatt F 2003 The contribution of parenting practices in a risk and resiliency model of children's adjustment. *British Journal of Developmental Psychology* 21:469–80.

Rowe J, Barnes M 2007 Families in transition: early parenting. In M McAllister (ed.), *Solution focused nursing. Rethinking practice*. Palgrave, Houndmills, UK, pp. 49–62.

Saggers S, Sims M 2005 Diversity: beyond the nuclear family. In M Poole, *Family: changing families and changing times*. Allen & Unwin, Sydney, pp. 66–87.

Spencer N 2000 Social gradients in child health: why do they occur and what can paediatricians do about them? *Ambulatory Child Health* 6:191–202.

Statistics New Zealand 2004 *New Zealand family and household projections 2001 (base)–2021*. Wellington. Available at www.stats.govt.nz/analytical-reports/nz-family/.

Statistics New Zealand 2006 *Census data*. Available at www.stats.govt.nz/census/default.htm.

Wright L, Leahey M 2005 *Nurses and families: a guide to family assessment and intervention*, 4th edn. FA Davis, Philadelphia.

Chapter 2

Developing programs for the child, young person and family

Gay Edgecombe and Karen McBride-Henry

Learning outcomes

Reading this chapter will help you to:

- understand what constitutes a program
- understand program planning and development
- understand how programs support government health policy
- understand how programs can impact on health outcomes for children, young people and families
- identify the role of key stakeholder groups in program development
- identify the knowledge and skills required for nurses and midwives to engage in program development
- understand program evaluation, and
- appreciate the importance of collaboration between related service systems and the key roles nurses and midwives can play for families by integrating their care.

Introduction

This chapter explores the development of healthcare programs for the child, young person and family, within the context of policy frameworks that guide national health priorities. The World Health Organization (WHO) defines a program as 'an organised aggregate of activities directed towards the attainment of defined objectives and targets' (1984a p. 4). These objectives and targets are generally expressed in terms of health policies or strategies established by international organisations, national and state governments, and regional health service providers. Programs are the frontline, or operational, mechanism through which we attempt to implement these policies; therefore, they must address policy aims while at the same time serving the target community.

Nurses and midwives working in the community have many opportunities to become involved in the public policy-making process that may lead to program development, program implementation and ongoing evaluation. The majority of nurses and midwives, however, are involved in translating policy into practice (Hennessy 2000 p. 1). A recent example of the key role nurses and midwives can play was the development of discharge protocols for midwives and maternal and child health nurses to ensure continuity of care for women during antenatal care, childbirth and discharge into a maternal and child health service. This work was carried out in Australia during 2003–04 by a multidisciplinary team of policy makers, maternal and child health nurses and midwives. The protocols were launched in Victoria in 2004 (Department of Human Services 2004 p. 1) and are now being used across the state by public hospitals and the Maternal and Child Health Service.

Many early childhood programs have been developed in New Zealand and Australia over the past decade, reflecting the integral role that successful early childhood policy has played in the development of new programs. See Table 2.1 for examples in both countries. These successes have been supported by evidence-based research (Lumley et al. 2003) and a response to informed community need (Keating & Hertzman 1999). This chapter explores program development as it relates to midwives and nurses working with children, young people and families. It discusses how government health policies set the context in which such programs exist, and presents a range of issues surrounding program planning and implementation, illustrated with examples drawn from the authors' experience in both Australia and New Zealand.

Table 2.1 Linking policy to program development

Policy	Government or sector level	Program
	New Zealand examples	
Ten steps to successful breastfeeding (World Health Organization & UNICEF 1989)	The Ministry of Health New Zealand consulted with key stakeholders and subsequently developed the *DHB tool kit: to improve nutrition* (2001a) to educate healthcare professionals about the Baby Friendly Hospital Initiative.	Different District Health Boards (DHBs) and small maternity hospitals began to develop strategies and programs to assist them in implementing the Baby Friendly Hospital Initiative.
Ottawa charter for health promotion (World Health Organization 1986)	The *Primary health care strategy* was created by the Ministry of Health New Zealand (2001b). Its key aims are to provide population-based healthcare and promote the role of the community in health promotion and preventive care. DHBs respond by adjusting organisation visions, and aligning planning and funding with the policy.	A Policy and Guidelines Group in a Child Health Service embrace a philosophy of 'seamless care', which emphasises integrated, interdisciplinary collaboration to improve healthcare delivery. This results in a program that crosses traditional tertiary and community healthcare boundaries (see Box 2.3 Practice highlight). *cont.*

Table 2.1 Linking policy to program development—*cont.*

Policy	Government or sector level	Program
	Australian examples	
Ottawa charter for health promotion (World Health Organization 1986)	In 1999, the new state government of Victoria planned to establish a secondary school nursing program with a strong emphasis on health promotion.	A new secondary school nursing program is implemented in 2000–01. Each school nurse is allocated two state-funded secondary schools. The following program goal illustrates the influence of the *Ottawa charter*. 'Goal 1: Play a key role in reducing negative health outcomes and risk-taking behaviours among young people, including drug and alcohol abuse, tobacco smoking, eating disorders, obesity, depression, suicide and injuries' (Department of Human Services 2000 p. 3).
Building healthy public policy is a goal of the *Ottawa charter* (look this up on the internet). Such policy is designed to integrate all aspects of the healthcare system providing services for families.	In 2003, the state government of Victoria established a working party to develop protocols for state maternity services and the state's Maternal and Child Health Service to assist the care of newborn infants and their families by improved discharge processes.	The protocols were published and distributed in 2004 to midwives (employed by midwifery programs) and maternal and child health nurses employed by Maternal and Child Health (MCH) programs. A key principle underlying the protocol is: '. . . enhance continuity of care for recent mothers and their babies from pregnancy through early parenthood, as provided by maternity and MCH services (this aim will be realised through improved care planning supported by effective communication and collaboration)' (Department of Human Services 2004 p. 1).

Setting the scene: a program development scenario

Developing and implementing healthcare programs generally relies on funding from a government agency, which implies that, if a proposed program is to proceed, it must be well supported at the state, regional, local government and/or national level. This is likely to be achieved only if the program is aligned with the priorities set out in current national or state/regional healthcare policy. However, it is important to recognise that effective policy development also requires input and support from frontline staff, which may be achieved, for example, through the participation of nurses and midwives in multidisciplinary teams.

Of course, securing funding is not the end of the story—staff involved in a program will face a range of difficulties before reaching a successful outcome. Currently, one of the most significant of these is the 'silo' culture that exists in child, young person and family health services. This refers to the tendency for different sectors, such as primary healthcare, early childhood education and mental healthcare, to provide the community with specialised services without communicating with each other. If you reflect on your current workplace, you will recognise the frustration this creates for the families you are working with, as they negotiate their way through early childhood services. You will be frustrated by not being able to obtain all the information you need from other early years professionals to assist your work with families.

We present a simple scenario describing some of the key players and issues surrounding policy and program development in the context of child, young person and family health, related to healthy eating and obesity. The example presented demonstrates the problems of silo culture and the potential of thinking outside the square of individual departments.

The nurse or midwife

You are attending a monthly community health meeting of all staff in your region who are involved in early childhood care. The speakers are working on a program proposal for the local health department designed to reduce the incidence of childhood obesity. You decide to volunteer because you are very concerned about the number of children in your maternal and health nursing practice who are overweight. A close friend of yours is also interested. She is the school nurse in the local secondary school and has introduced a number of programs in her school designed to reduce obesity and prevent type 2 diabetes. You had not previously considered becoming involved in program development, because you thought such work was only undertaken by managers and policy makers from the health department.

The program proposal team

A multidisciplinary team is working on a program proposal related to childhood obesity, which has been increasing at an alarming rate over the past 10 years. Governments in a number of countries have recognised an urgent need to act. The team lacks sufficient input from frontline clinicians and is pleased that several nurses and midwives are keen to review the draft program proposal and provide feedback.

Program silo: nurses and midwives

Child and family nurses Elizabeth and Rani are concerned that their roles are becoming less relevant as childhood health services evolve. Their view is that: 'We are always the ones left holding the baby. We must argue that some of the new childhood obesity funding should come our way in the form of additional staff, so we can spend more time with families working on childhood obesity prevention. Our program is designed to work with families for at least the first 5 years of the child's life. What is the point in giving this program to agencies that do not understand child development?'

Program silo: policy makers

Ted and Bruce are involved in policy development at a regional health office, and are worried about the 'silo culture' associated with early childhood services. Ted is frustrated, and comments that 'health services don't talk to education services, the child and family nurses don't work with the early childhood teachers, and the midwives do their thing and so on. They all do their own thing. How can we get them to work together on childhood obesity?'

Integrated programs: nurses and midwives

Farrokh and Ilsa are maternal and child health nurses working in an enhanced home-visiting program targeted to meet the needs of vulnerable families. They are pleased with the integrated aspects of their work. Their view is that: 'We feel so supported in our practice. We have a great multidisciplinary team and the clinical supervision helps us keep up to date with best practice.' Both have attended team meetings to plan for the introduction of a childhood obesity prevention initiative.

Integrated programs: policy makers

Bruce, a senior policy maker in the regional health office, is excited by the maternal and child health enhanced home-visiting program, and suggests to Ted that it could serve as the platform from which to deliver the childhood obesity initiative.

It might be useful at this point to map the people, organisations and policy and service levels involved in the scenario presented to develop a picture of the complexities of program development.

The next section examines health policy and its impact on program development. Policy makers in Australia and New Zealand are working closely with their existing early childhood programs to introduce programs designed to prevent and reduce population health problems such as childhood obesity.

Health policy and its effect on program development

Any regional child and family health program in Australia and New Zealand exists within the context of global and national health policies, which tend to determine health priorities such as reducing childhood obesity. While these factors may be quite removed from their day-to-day activities, nurses and midwives need to understand that they have a significant influence on health priorities, and the availability of funding for services, at regional and local levels.

Therefore, when proposing or establishing any program, consideration must be given to the relevant health policies that support it. For infants, children and young people, early intervention is vital. Therefore, it is also important to review the principles of health promotion, as prevention and early intervention represents the core practice of child and family nurses. This guidance is particularly important when planning to manage major public health issues such as childhood obesity. The following original principles of health promotion were prepared by a World Health Organization (WHO) working party (1984b p. 20) and remain an excellent starting point:

'1. *Health promotion involves the population as a whole in the context of their everyday life, rather than focusing on people at risk for specific diseases.* It enables people to take control over, and responsibility for, their health as an important component of everyday life, both as spontaneous and organized action for health. This requires full and continuing access to information about health and how it might be sought by *all* the population, using, therefore, all dissemination methods available.

2. *Health promotion is directed towards action on the determinants or causes of health.* Health promotion, therefore, requires a close cooperation of sectors beyond health services, reflecting the diversity of conditions that influence health. Government, at both local and national levels, has a unique responsibility to act appropriately in a timely way to ensure that the 'total' environment, which is beyond the control of individuals and groups, is conducive to health.

3. *Health promotion combines diverse, but complementary, methods or approaches,* including communication, education, legislation, fiscal measures, organizational change, community development and spontaneous local activities against health hazards.

4. *Health promotion aims particularly at effective and concrete public participation.* This focus requires the further development of problem-defining and decision-making life skills, both individually and collectively.

5. While health promotion is basically an activity in the health and social fields, and not a medical service, *health professionals—particularly in primary health care—have an important role in nurturing and enabling health promotion.* Health professionals should work outwards, developing their special contributions in education and health advocacy' (emphasis in original).

More recently, the scope for nurses to enable populations not only at the coalface of healthcare delivery but also through participation in policy and service development is gathering momentum. Edelman and Mandle (2006 p. 613) are of the view that nurses need to consider three principal goals with respect to health promotion:

'1. Participate in health promotion policy development.

2. Influence public expectations about health promotion.

3. Promote equitable access to preventive health care.'

These principles underpin global, national and local policies, which in turn inform program development.

The global perspective

Global health organisations such as the WHO and the United Nations Children's Fund (UNICEF) provide guidance on global health issues, which informs the decision makers in individual countries who are responsible for setting health priorities and policies. These organisations attempt to focus the attention of individual nations on healthcare issues that are considered to be of the utmost importance from a global perspective.

For example, the United Nations Convention on the Rights of the Child or UNCROC (1990 article 24) states that supporting nations must 'recognise the rights of the child to the enjoyment of the highest attainable standard of health and to facilities for the treatment of illness and rehabilitation'. It also states that governments should ensure that children be given the right to access appropriate healthcare, which means that governments must embrace this right when planning child and family health policy at a national level. An example of the flow-through of prioritisation at a global level to national policy and service initiatives is set out in Box 2.1.

Health literacy is an aspect of policy and program development that also filters through global, national and program levels to be relevant in the everyday work of nurses with families. Leaders in the field are providing useful global challenges for us all. For example, Nutbeam and Kickbusch (2000 p. 183) provide guidance in their editorial, 'Advancing health literacy: a global challenge for the 21st century'. They argue for the need to ensure that people have access to education in order 'to improve the health literacy of persons with inadequate or marginal literacy skills'.

Going beyond the notion of information dissemination, health literacy seeks to achieve more than information dissemination. Rather, it seeks to increase the accessibility of information and motivation for engaging in health-seeking behaviours. This is an issue that nurses and midwives deal with daily in New Zealand and Australia in our multicultural communities.

The national perspective

New Zealand and Australia both have national mechanisms for developing policy and programs. Box 2.1 gives an example of how global policy influences national policy and planning in regard to breastfeeding programs in New Zealand. Understanding national planning pathways is central to program development. An outline of healthcare organisation for each country is now provided with a specific focus on child health policy development.

New Zealand

The New Zealand government plans and directs the provision of healthcare for its citizens through the Ministry of Health (MOH NZ), which is charged with implementing health-related legislation, such as the New Zealand Public Health and Disability Act (Ministry of Health New Zealand 2000b), and the development of nation-wide health strategies and policy. Policy development at the MOH NZ takes into account the recommendations of the WHO and other international organisations, with child healthcare direction based on documents such as the UNCROC.

Box 2.1 Practice highlight: applying global policy—national programs for promoting breastfeeding in New Zealand

Global policy

In 1990, WHO and UNICEF produced the *Innocenti declaration: breastfeeding in the 1990s—a global treatise* (World Health Organization & UNICEF 1990). It aimed to promote breastfeeding globally, enable women to practise exclusive breastfeeding and to pressure governments to implement policies that would support women to breastfeed. The declaration argued the optimal nutritive qualities of breastfeeding for growth and development, its role in reducing infant morbidity and mortality, enhancing women's health, and producing economic benefits. It stipulated exclusive breastfeeding for all infants to 6 months of age and that breastfeeding be maintained to age 2.

The declaration sets out targets for individual countries to achieve, and strategies to help meet targets. These include:

1. the appointment of a national breastfeeding coordinator
2. the establishment of a multisector national breastfeeding committee
3. ensuring hospitals support the '10 steps to successful breastfeeding', and
4. compliance with the 'International code for the marketing of breast-milk substitutes', and legislation to protect breastfeeding women.

National policy

In New Zealand, the Department of Health (now called the Ministry of Health) signalled its support for the *Innocenti declaration* (Gordon 1998, Vogel & Mitchell 1998) and a meeting was convened in 1991 to reconsider the code's place within New Zealand. Little unifying action was taken. In 1999, the Ministry of Health established clear breastfeeding definitions and, in 2002, established national breastfeeding targets and a breastfeeding action plan (Ministry of Health New Zealand 2002).

Programs

In 1992, a 'breastfeeding kit' was developed by the then health department to educate healthcare professionals about the code for breast-milk substitutes and the *Innocenti declaration*. In 1998, the New Zealand Breastfeeding Authority (n.d.) was established to coordinate the many breastfeeding stakeholders and oversee the Baby Friendly Hospital Initiative (see Ch 6 for more information), a program promoted by WHO and known to increase breastfeeding rates.

Outstanding issues

1. A national breastfeeding coordinator has never been appointed.
2. No legislation requiring compliance with the code has been developed and, while monitored, compliance remains voluntary.
3. Breastfeeding rates have shown little change in the last decade.

A number of key national strategies have a significant effect on healthcare provision for children and their families in New Zealand. These include the *Child health strategy* (Ministry of Health New Zealand 1998), which was introduced in Chapter 1, the *New Zealand health strategy* (Ministry of Health New Zealand 2000a), and the *Primary health care strategy* (Ministry of Health New Zealand 2001b). These documents highlight the nation's healthcare goals and the directions for care provision, looking forward some 10 years from the date of publication.

The vision for children's healthcare set out in *Child health strategy* is 'our children / tamariki: seen, heard and getting what they need' (p. vii). The strategy outlines a number of guiding principles for the development of child health programs in New Zealand, including:

1. children's needs are paramount
2. childcare services should be based on 'international best practice, research and education' (p. 19), and
3. childcare services should be culturally acceptable and safe.

It also acknowledges that services require regular review to ensure they continue to meet the changing needs of children and families.

The *New Zealand health strategy* is based on similar principles, but highlights the special relationship between Maori and the Crown under the Treaty of Waitangi. It lays out a number of health objectives, based on emergent health determinants, which include improving nutrition, increasing the level of physical activity, reducing obesity, improving oral health, and reducing community violence.

The *Primary health care strategy* identifies six key goals that include working with local communities, identifying and removing health inequalities, improving access to comprehensive services so that health can be improved, maintained and restored, the coordination of care across services, workforce development, and continuous quality improvement.

All of these policy documents provide direction to regional District Health Boards (DHBs), which plan and distribute funding for health services at the regional and local levels.

Australia

The Australian federal government shares responsibility for health services with the states and territories. The two key federal government departments involved with child health and parenting are the Department of Health and Ageing and the Department of Families, Community Services and Indigenous Affairs. A number of other national bodies also influence child health policy and parenting, including the Australian Research Alliance for Children and Youth, the National Health and Medical Research Council and the Australian Institute of Family Studies.

However, it is important to note that the consideration of child health issues is not restricted to health and community service agencies. Australian governments at the national, state and local levels all recognise the need to consider children and their families when developing any new policies or programs. For example, policy related to road safety integrates research findings on road accidents involving children; similarly, policy on juvenile justice incorporates knowledge of the factors that contribute to young people coming into conflict with the law.

As in New Zealand, Australian governments and key stakeholders in child health policy development are in close contact with global organisations such as the WHO, the World Bank, the International Council of Nurses (ICN), and key national centres for child health in other countries, such as the Canadian Institute of Child Health. Both New Zealand and Australian child health and parenting experts have served on committees for global agencies such as the WHO. A number of global policies and programs are recognised annually. An example is World Breastfeeding Week.

In a review of child health policy in Australia, Liu et al. (2004 p. 3) found that the most frequently targeted child health issues are nutrition, Indigenous health, immunisation, general health, tobacco and drug issues, early years, child protection, physical activity, screening and surveillance, injury and mental health. This list does not include childhood obesity because, at the time the study was done, only one state had developed specific policies for it. However, the study's authors noted that the document *Healthy weight 2008: Australia's future. The national agenda for young people and their families* (Australian Health Ministers Conference 2003) was being disseminated across the country. Since then, policies and programs for childhood obesity have been under development across Australia.

Embedded in the Australian national child health policy (National Public Health Partnership 2005) introduced in Chapter 1 are key initiatives for improving child health and wellbeing, and are central to program development. Their intent is to develop:

» national evidence-based guidelines for antenatal care
» a consistent and cross-sectoral national approach for identifying and supporting vulnerable families in the antenatal period and early years
» child health and wellbeing indicators, and
» core, common child health and wellbeing competencies for all who deliver care to children (National Public Health Partnership 2005).

The local perspective

National policy provides guidance in New Zealand for DHBs and in Australia for state and local government and regional health authorities when planning service delivery and the distribution of funding. This assists them in ensuring that program support and development are aligned with the nation's healthcare goals. However, local demographics and health determinants are important influences at the local level that affect program development and uptake by individual DHBs (in New Zealand) or local government authorities and regionalised health services (in Australia). These are the factors that might first impress nurses and midwives in their everyday practice and are most likely to influence them when they are developing child and family health programs at the local level.

Developing programs

So what does the policy-making process and subsequent program development look like? Diers (2004 p. 153) reports that 'the policy-making process is generally outlined as getting on the agenda or agenda setting, policy formulation, policy implementation, policy evaluation, and modification'.

Research by Edgecombe (1992) examined the role that child and family nurses played in these processes in one Australian state over several decades (from the 1950s). See Box 2.2 and Figure 2.1 for a brief overview of the findings and the application

Box 2.2 Research highlight: critical ingredients for program development

Research by Edgecombe (1992) examined the public policy-making process and aspects of program development and program implementation in a state-wide community health nursing service. The study found that a number of critical ingredients were required for the development of successful policy and its subsequent program development. These ingredients were needs, vision, support, patron, structure and funding (see Fig 2.1).

Figure 2.1 Public policy process and program development

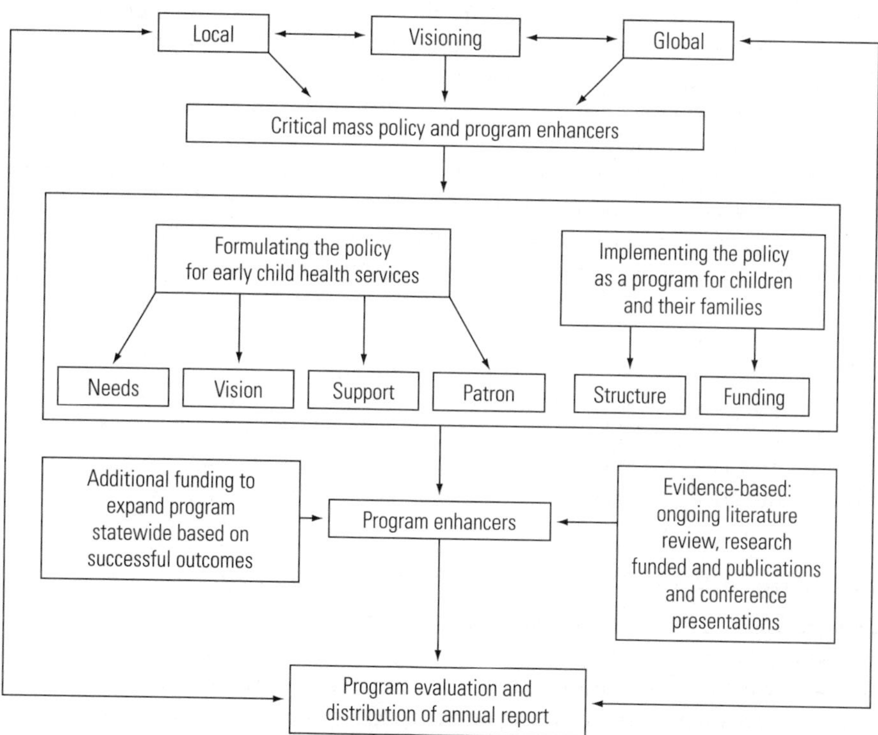

Source: Adapted from G Edgecombe 1992 Critical ingredients for public policy: a study of public health nursing policy process in Western Australia. Unpublished thesis, University of Western Australia, p. 381.

of the research in practice. Policy processes are not linear. Some aspects of the policy process take place simultaneously, while other policy processes may take years before a program is eventually developed and implemented. Nurses and midwives were involved in many aspects of the policy process, program development and implementation and program evaluation.

Since 1992, the author has used this knowledge to develop policy documents such as the *Maternal and child health service program standards* (Edgecombe et al. 1995) and the *Secondary school nursing program standards* (Edgecombe & Ward 2006). She is also using this information when teaching about the policy-making processes in her courses and for examining existing policy processes such as the Australian federal government's Council of Australian Governments (COAG) 2006–2207 exploration of the need for new policies related to early childhood development: see www.coag.gov.au/meetings/100206/index.htm#reform. For example, who and what is involved with the policy process elements: needs, vision, support, patron, structure and funding.

There are a number of processes that must be undertaken prior to establishing any healthcare program. The link between global and national policy as these relate to services has been set out above; recall the development of breastfeeding initiatives in New Zealand set out in Box 2.1. Consider also UNCROC, which highlights the importance of a national immunisation program, which is, in turn, reflected in national strategy (see also Ch 7).

The importance of understanding this link or dynamic between global, national and local is critical to planning any health program that targets child and family health. In the following section we present a set of principles to guide the establishment of a nursing or midwifery program. Box 2.3 demonstrates the application of the principles in a New Zealand program.

The prescription of EpiPens for children who have experienced an anaphylactic reaction at a large regional children's hospital was identified as problematic, as significant issues around follow-up care were evident. Post-discharge support for these children and their families was fragmented, with responsibility for ongoing care spread across a range of service providers, each operating largely on its own. This resulted in a lack of consistent care being offered to these children and their families; therefore, a practice development group was formed with the purpose of developing a clinical practice guideline that would support seamless care for children being discharged from hospital with a prescription for an EpiPen. The aim of the group was to establish a fully integrated care-delivery system that facilitates a smooth transition from acute to community-based care.

Identifying and responding to community needs

A crucial prerequisite for establishing any program is an understanding of the community the program will serve, with emphasis on its health needs. That is, start local. This will typically require a community needs analysis, which examines health inequalities, population distribution and demographics. Of particular interest is the number and percentage of children in an area, average household income, ethnic make-up, avoidable hospital admission rates, infectious disease rates, reported violence rates, as well as morbidity and mortality data. In addition, knowledge of all available primary and secondary health services is important. This information provides essential insight into the health service gaps within the community.

For example, if you wanted to develop a targeted program for women who wish to breastfeed within a certain geographical area, there are a number of ways that community need could be assessed. To begin with, it is important to know which women are most likely to breastfeed, and what modifiable factors impact on breastfeeding rates. Extensive literature searching for research on successful breastfeeding initiatives is a useful exercise. It is also important to assess what services are available in specific geographic areas that support and promote breastfeeding,

Box 2.3 Practice highlight: program development for children requiring EpiPens

In 2001, the Ministry of Health New Zealand released the *Primary health care strategy* (2001b). In part, this policy was developed with the aim of building healthcare capacity and health promotion in keeping with the *Ottawa charter for health promotion* (World Health Organization 1986). The strategy outlined a vision for the advancement of primary healthcare services throughout New Zealand. Its primary goal was to provide population-based healthcare through community health promotion and preventive care; however, achieving these will require many changes to current healthcare delivery structures, which favours tertiary-based healthcare.

Identifying and responding to community needs

The need to transition services into the community environment prompted the formation of a group, within a child health service of a regional DHB, to tackle the issue of care for children who required EpiPens following an anaphylactic reaction.

Promoting the idea

The group identified the current care providers and convened a meeting of concerned stakeholders, including external agencies such as public health agencies, general practitioners, telephone companies, and Work and Income New Zealand. These meetings resulted in identifying the need for care coordinators who would oversee the management of affected children through the various health service providers and external commercial agencies.

Program implementation

An appropriate care coordination group, the Paediatric Nursing Service, which spanned the interface between acute and community care, was nominated to oversee the care of these children. It agreed to:

- provide families with an initial home visit for support and education on both EpiPens and anaphylaxis
- act as a liaison between the family and its primary healthcare provider, to establish ongoing support and education and facilitate renewal of prescriptions as needed
- for children under 5 years of age, initiate education programs within either the daycare or kindergarten setting as needed, and
- for children over 5 years of age, provide a referral to the Public Health Service for a school-based education program.

Program evaluation

This guideline development program has led to a significant improvement in the quality of care, by eliminating unnecessary delays and ensuring that all required services are delivered at the appropriate time. This development serves to demonstrate how seamless care can facilitate program development and enhance child and family health outcomes. It has provided an opportunity for children and their families, affected by anaphylaxis, to gain control over their health. This is in keeping with the health promoting principles outlined by the WHO (1986) in the *Ottawa charter*, which asserts that health promotion needs to focus on giving families increased control over their health and its associated determinants.

while also identifying which factors undermine and inhibit breastfeeding. Having conversations with those working with breastfeeding women will also assist in identifying salient issues. In addition, holding focus groups with breastfeeding women will also assist with the identification of factors that impact the region.

There are a number of well-known research methods that have been developed to aid in identifying and responding to community needs (Clendon 2004–05, Rigby et al. 2003, Shupe et al. 2000). These include literature reviews, focus groups and community surveys. Reviewing the effectiveness of existing programs may also help in assessing the appropriateness of the planned program.

Promoting the idea

After the needs analysis has been completed, it would be useful to assemble a team of people with an interest in the program. The team would ideally consist of representatives from the health, education and social services sectors who are invested in the community and have a working knowledge of community strengths and potential service gaps. From this position, the team can assist in establishing objectives, around which a well-targeted program can be developed.

The program team can also contribute to an appropriate action plan, a realistic budget and the identification of local stakeholders. The last point is especially important, as having strong relationships with key community members is essential for program promotion, and will assist in gauging the level of support for a program within the wider community. For example, if you are seeking to develop a breastfeeding promotion program, it would be beneficial to develop strong relationships with the community and other key stakeholders such as appropriate women's community groups, community leaders, early childhood education providers, public health nurses, maternal and child health nurses, Plunket nurses, school nurses and local general practitioners. They will assist you to understand the local culture and provide insight into appropriate community venues for the program's promotion. Need is a complex concept, grounded in objective data but mediated in the everyday world of a community, thus making understanding and responsiveness critical early activities for those hoping to provide relevant and acceptable services.

Gaining community support requires that the community actively contribute to program development, a process referred to as the community partnership model. The importance of community partnership in proposed health programs has been highlighted by many nursing and midwifery researchers (Claeson & Waldman 2000, Clendon 2004–05, Fraenkel 2006, Lee et al. 2003). This concept can easily be incorporated as a fundamental philosophical tenet in any program; without it, community-focused initiatives will have limited success (Clendon 2004–05, Fraenkel 2006, Lee et al. 2003).

Program implementation

Implementing a healthcare program will require that a number of operational issues be addressed. Early steps may include documentation of the program's policies and procedures, such as the processes for tracking client progress and the mechanisms for program evaluation. Infrastructure requirements also need to be considered, which may include provision of computers and associated networks and software, office space and screening equipment to name just a few.

Community members may have working knowledge of existing resources and their input on the location for a program will be invaluable. Media campaigns may also be needed to publicise the program's launch, or in some cases to assist in establishing community support. If you have been working with the local community to establish a program, such as the breastfeeding promotion program, then this will assist greatly in the implementation of the program.

Workforce development is another key aspect of program implementation. Providing sufficient training to enable staff to obtain the clinical skills to successfully deliver interventions aimed at promoting health and wellness for children and their families is of the utmost importance. Sharing the health promotion principles that underpin the program that has been developed will provide vision and help emphasise the importance of the program. Using the breastfeeding promotion program as an example, awareness of global policies such as '10 steps to successful breastfeeding' (World Health Organization & UNICEF 1989) and the *Innocenti declaration* (World Health Organization & UNICEF 1990) would help staff understand and support the program to be implemented at the local level. Staff also need to be aware of the local policies and procedures that underpin the program, and keep up to date on changes to these. Box 2.4 provides a practical activity that will help you to develop insights from the coalface of program development.

Box 2.4 Critical questions and reflections: finding out more about program development

Interview a person with whom you work who has been involved in the development of a new program for families with young children or for young people. Ask about the processes they were involved in to develop the program. Make a list of the stages, processes and techniques they used to successfully implement the program. What worked and what did not work?

Program evaluation

Historically, nurses and midwives have conducted a wide range of exciting, innovative programs; however, these have often been set up without appropriate mechanisms for evaluating health outcomes, in this way undermining a program's effectiveness. It is important that an effective evaluation mechanism be built into any program from the outset. Common evaluation tools include surveys, fourth generation evaluation (see Guba & Lincoln 1989), the DEEP tool (see Walsh et al. 2005), statistical information on the types of clients accessing the program, consumer focus groups and key stakeholder interviews.

A particularly useful tool during an evaluation cycle is the client or patient satisfaction survey. Well-developed patient satisfaction surveys can provide important information about how children and their families experience the service (see Hill 1997 and Mills et al. 2003). They can also provide valuable insights into operational issues, such as the usefulness of program venues or associated materials.

The collection of evaluation data must be well thought through ahead of time, so that the information collected will give maximum benefit. Data should be stored in a way that facilitates access and subsequent analysis, which will involve the development of administrative processes to support the program right from the start.

Many policy documents provide guidance on program development processes (e.g. *A guide to developing public health programmes: a generic programme logic model*, published in 2006 by the New Zealand MOH). Some universities offer the services of research statisticians who can evaluate approaches to data collection and analysis at minimal cost, which may be invaluable during the planning phase of program evaluation.

Ideally, work with the local research centre set up for child and family research. Such centres are usually linked to or based within a university and provide regular research seminars where research findings are presented. A large research team has recently evaluated an Australian project called 'Evaluation of the stronger families and communities strategy 2000–04'. As part of the evaluation an issues paper was prepared, titled *Early intervention—particularly in early childhood* (Rogers et al. 2004). This paper can be accessed at www.facs.gov.au/internet/facsinternet.nsf/aboutfacs/programs/sfsc-early_intervention.htm. This website contains other documents related to the evaluation, including newsletters explaining the evaluation.

Managing change

New child health polices and programs are being developed in Australia and New Zealand, and will change aspects of midwifery and child and family nursing practice. Nurses and midwives in both countries have a long history of effectively adapting their practice to meet family needs. However, change can be difficult to manage if it has not been carefully considered during policy and program development. Successful programs have considered the effects of change on the people involved throughout the development process, recognising that keeping people informed of changes and the reasons why change is occurring is crucial to effective change management.

Ford et al. (2004) argue the need for change to be managed through a process of participative-democratic practices, which involves three distinct principles: 'creating space for new communicative interaction, safe-guarding a credible and open process and reclaiming suppressed views' (p. 21). Creating space for communication means prioritising opportunities to communicate how changes will occur. Safe-guarding processes involves dealing with the difficult issues and developing action plans to deal with them as they arise. Finally, reclaiming suppressed views involves taking the time to listen to concerns about former processes, and incorporating solutions into the future program planning. Stripped down, this change process means involving staff in the process of change through transparent lines of communication between those directing change and those who are being affected by the change.

It is important that nurses and midwives are involved in all aspects of program development—from the formation of policy, to locally embedded practice development initiatives. Historically, we have taken a back seat in driving such initiatives, instead taking our lead from other professional groups. It is important to harness the knowledge we have gained through working alongside communities, and use this to shape policy and subsequent development of programs. In addition to this, we also need to become active change agents through practice development methodologies, which require us to focus on achievable, community-centred initiatives. In these actions we will create sustainable and useful programs, which are based upon appropriate health promoting principles. Box 2.5 provides an activity that will assist you to apply the concepts presented.

Box 2.5 Critical questions and reflections: a program proposal

1. Think about examples from your practice where a specific nursing program could improve child, young people and family health outcomes.
2. Think about child health policy in your country and region, and how it might relate to the development of your proposed program.
3. What issues would you need to address to make the program a reality?
4. How might you evaluate the proposed program?

Conclusion

Nurses and midwives in Australia and New Zealand have a long history of involvement in developing and running programs to improve health outcomes for children, young people and families. This process is, by necessity, strongly informed by global and national policy, which drives healthcare priorities and the availability of funding for programs. The case studies and examples explored in this chapter have illustrated the need to address policy considerations during program development, while at the same time meeting the needs of local communities.

Guiding principles for developing healthcare programs have also been discussed in this chapter, as has the need to develop tools to effectively evaluate how programs contribute to enhanced health outcomes for children, young people and their families. This chapter has also highlighted the importance of creating structures that provide flexibility, so programs continue to meet the needs of children, young people and their families.

Key points

» Consult widely about programs for children and young people.
» Know the work and follow the work of national and international leaders in your field.
» Be familiar with the global and national policies that impact on children, young people and their families.
» Know the health goals and targets for children, young people and their families in your country and others.
» Develop relationships with members of the community in which programs will be implemented.
» Attend key conferences related to program management.
» Embed continuous quality improvement in any program.
» Engage in practice development to achieve excellence in clinical care provision.

» Have a strategic plan for implementing change.
» Build in program evaluation from day one.

Useful resources

There are numerous websites that provide information about programs for children, young people and families. A selection of these appears below:

» www.plunket.org.nz/Index2.htm
» www.dhs.vic.gov.au/commcare
» www.dhs.vic.gov.au/earlychood
» www.paediatrics.org.nz/
» www.kidshealth.org.nz/
» www.cyh.com/Default.aspx?p=1
» www.aifs.gov.au/institute/links.html

Health promotion links include:

» www.who.int/hpr/health.promotion.shtml
» http://whqlibdoc.who.int/euro/-1993/ICP_HSR_602_m01.pdf

References

Australian Health Ministers Conference 2003 *Healthy weight 2008: Australia's future. The national agenda for young people and their families*. National Obesity Taskforce Secretariat, Department of Health and Ageing, Canberra.

Claeson M, Waldman R 2000 The evolution of child health programs in developing countries: from targeting diseases to targeting people. *Bulletin of the World Health Organization* 78(10):1234–45.

Clendon J 2004–05 Demonstrating outcomes in a nurse-led clinic: how primary health care nurses make a difference to children and their families. *Contemporary Nurse* 18(1–2):164–76.

Department of Human Services (DHS) 2000 Victorian secondary school nursing program: consultation paper. DHS, Melbourne.

Department of Human Services (DHS) 2004 *Continuity of care: a communication protocol for Victorian public maternity services and the Maternal and Child Health Service.* Community Care Division, Victorian Government Department of Human Services, Melbourne. Available at www.health.vic.gov.au/maternitycare/.

Diers D 2004 *Speaking of nursing . . . narratives of practice, research, policy and the profession*. Jones and Bartlett Publishers, Sudbury, Massachusetts.

Edelman CL, Mandle CL 2006 *Health promotion throughout the lifespan*, 6th edn. Elsevier Mosby, St Louis, Missouri.

Edgecombe G 1992 Critical ingredients for public policy: a study of public health nursing policy process in Western Australia. Unpublished thesis, University of Western Australia.

Edgecombe GA, Mackey R, Hindell A et al. 1995 *Maternal and child health service program standards*. Health and Community Services, Melbourne.

Edgecombe G, Ward M 2006 *Secondary school nursing program standards*. Office for Children, Juvenile Justice and Youth Services Branch, Secondary School

Nursing Program, Department of Human Services, Melbourne.
Ford R, Boss W, Angermeier I et al. 2004 Adapting to change in health care: aligning strategic intent and operational capacity. *Hospital Topics: Research and Perspectives on Healthcare* 82(4):20–9.
Fraenkel P 2006 Engaging families as experts: collaborative family programme development. *Family Process* 42(2):237–57.
Gordon R 1998 The role of La Leche League in the promotion and support of breastfeeding. In A Beasley & A Trlin (eds), *Breastfeeding in New Zealand: practice, problems and policy*. Dunmore Press, Palmerston North, pp. 127–39.
Guba E, Lincoln Y 1989 *Fourth generation evaluation*. Sage Publications, London.
Hennessy D 2000 The emerging themes. In D Hennessy & P Spurgeon (eds), *Health policy and nursing*. Macmillan Press, London.
Hill J 1997 Patient satisfaction in a nurse-led rheumatology clinic. *Journal of Advanced Nursing* 25:347–54.
Keating DP, Hertzman C 1999 Modernity's paradox. In D Keating & C Hertzman (eds), *Developmental health and the wealth of nations*. Guildford Press, New York, pp. 1–7.
Lee A, Tsang C, Lee S, To C 2003 A comprehensive 'healthy schools programme' to promote school health: the Hong Kong experience in joining the efforts of health and education sectors. *Journal of Epidemiological Community Health* 57:174–7.
Liu M, Mead C, Green J 2004 *An audit of child public health related policies in Australia*. National Public Health Partnership, Melbourne.
Lumley J, Brown S, Gunn J 2003 Getting research transfer into policy and practice in maternity care. In V Lin & B Gibson (eds), *Evidence-based health policy*. Oxford University Press, Melbourne, pp. 272–97.
Mills K, Penny N, Power R, Mercey D 2003 Comparing doctor- and nurse-led care in a sexual health clinic: patient satisfaction questionnaire. *Journal of Advanced Nursing* 42(1):64–72.
Ministry of Health New Zealand (MOH NZ) 1998 *Child health strategy*. Available at www.moh.govt.nz/moh.nsf/wpg_Index/Publications-Index.
Ministry of Health New Zealand (MOH NZ) 2000a *The New Zealand health strategy*. MOH NZ, Wellington. Available at www.maorihealth.govt.nz/moh.nsf/pagesma/4/$File/NZHthStrat.pdf.
Ministry of Health New Zealand (MOH NZ) 2000b *The New Zealand Public Health and Disability Act*. Available at www.moh.govt.nz/moh.nsf/wpg_Index/Publications-Index.
Ministry of Health New Zealand (MOH NZ) 2001a *DHB tool kit: to improve nutrition*. MOH NZ, Wellington.
Ministry of Health New Zealand (MOH NZ) 2001b *The primary health care strategy*. Available at www.moh.govt.nz/moh.nsf/wpg_Index/Publications-Index.
Ministry of Health New Zealand (MOH NZ) 2002 *Breastfeeding: a guide to action*. MOH NZ, Wellington. Available at www.moh.govt.nz.
Ministry of Health New Zealand (MOH NZ) 2006 *A guide to developing public health programmes: a generic programme logic model*. Available at www.moh.govt.nz/moh.nsf/wpg_Index/Publications-Index
National Public Health Partnership 2005 *Healthy children: strengthening promotion and prevention across Australia. National Public Health Strategic Framework for*

Children 2005–2008. Available at www.dhs.vic.gov.au/nphp/workprog/chip/cyhactionplanbg.htm.

New Zealand Breastfeeding Authority n.d. Available at www.babyfriendly.org.nz/. Accessed 16 February 2007.

Nutbeam D, Kickbusch I 2000 Advancing health literacy: a global challenge for the 21st century. *Health Promotion International* 15(3):183–4.

Rigby M, Lennart K, Blair M, Metchler R 2003 Child health indicators for Europe: a priority for a caring society. *Child Health Indicators for Europe* 13(3):38–46.

Rogers P, Edgecombe G, Kimberley S et al. 2004 *Early intervention—particularly in early childhood. Evaluation of the Stronger Families and Communities Strategy 2000–04*. Department of Family and Community Services, Canberra. Available at www.facs.gov.au/internet/facsinternet.nsf/aboutfacs/programs/sfsc-early_intervention.htm.

Shupe A, Smith A, Stout C, McLaughlin H 2000 The importance of local data in unintended pregnancy prevention programming. *Maternal and Child Health Journal* 4(3):209–14.

United Nations Convention on the Rights of the Child (UNCROC) 1990. Available at www.unhchr.ch/html/menu3/b/k2crc.htm.

Vogel A, Mitchell E 1998 The baby friendly hospital initiative: evidence and implementation. In A Beasley & A Trlin (eds), *Breastfeeding in New Zealand: practice, problems and policy*. Dunmore Press, Palmerston North, pp. 169–92.

Walsh K, Lawless J, Moss C, Allbon C 2005 The development of an engagement tool for practice development. *Practice Development in Health Care* 4(3):124–30.

World Health Organization (WHO) 1984a *Glossary of terms used in the 'health for all' series, numbers 1–8*. WHO, Geneva

World Health Organization (WHO) 1984b *Health promotion: concepts and principles*. Report of a Working Group, 9–13 July. WHO Regional Office for Europe, Copenhagen. Available at http://whqlibdoc.who.int/euro/-1993/ICP_HSR_602_m01.pdf. Accessed 3 January 2007.

World Health Organization (WHO) 1986 *Ottawa charter for health promotion*. WHO, Geneva.

World Health Organization (WHO), UNICEF 1989 *Protecting, promoting and supporting breast-feeding: the special role of maternity services*. WHO, Geneva.

World Health Organization (WHO), UNICEF 1990 *The Innocenti declaration: breastfeeding in the 1990s—a global treatise*. WHO, Geneva.

Chapter 3

Towards partnership: Indigenous health in Australia and New Zealand

Sue Kruske, Evelyn Hikuroa and Vicki Bradford

Learning outcomes

Reading this chapter will help you to:

- » identify the key health issues affecting Aboriginal and Torres Strait Islander peoples and Maori
- » identify existing social, economic and political processes that contribute to inequalities in health between Indigenous and non-Indigenous peoples
- » understand the principles of cultural safety and their importance for healthcare for Indigenous people
- » distinguish between Indigenous peoples and ethnic minorities
- » discuss the impact of colonisation on the health of Indigenous peoples with specific reference to Australia and New Zealand, and
- » recognise the role of nursing in improving health outcomes for Indigenous peoples.

Introduction

Effective nursing or midwifery care requires an understanding of some of the key factors that influence the health of Indigenous peoples and their access to health services.[1]

1 To show respect to these populations when referring to Aboriginal Australians, Torres Strait Islander peoples and Maori as Indigenous peoples, Indigenous is capitalised.

There is misunderstanding and lack of awareness among non-Indigenous communities concerning Indigenous peoples, their health and healthcare. Education is at the heart of change in this situation. Traditionally, education systems have reflected the cultural dominance of the largest and most powerful group in society. This chapter therefore aims to assist students and practising nurses and midwives to recognise the role they play as members of the nursing or midwifery profession, and the wider health system, in providing safe, high-quality care to Indigenous families.

In this chapter, the significance of social history as it establishes current patterns of Indigenous health and illness, and of healthcare response, is argued as a significant principle and beginning point to a new awareness and understanding. The health issues for Indigenous children, young people and their families are rooted not only in the historical events of colonisation, but also in the ongoing social, economic and political processes that continue to marginalise Indigenous peoples and deny them the right to control their own affairs (self-determination).

While some health professionals, including nurses and midwives, do not see the relevance or significance of colonial history, others do. Understanding the historical experiences of Aboriginal and Torres Strait Islander peoples and Maori is a first step in critical education for change. While this genera peoples tion is not responsible for the past, change must be made in the present, as we are all responsible for the future. Given these premises, the reader is invited to engage critically and thoughtfully with the insights in this chapter and to consider not only the lingering impact of colonisation on the health of Indigenous peoples in Australia and New Zealand, but also ultimately the implications for nursing practice and health service delivery.

Definitions

The *Macquarie Dictionary* defines 'Indigenous' as 'originating in and characterising a particular region or country'. The term 'Indigenous' has been identified as problematic for some writers due to its general application to any country or land. This lack of specific acknowledgment of the Australian context diminishes their Aboriginality (New South Wales Health 2004). Therefore, where possible, this chapter uses the term 'Aboriginal and Torres Strait Islander peoples' to refer to the diversity of languages, cultural practices and spiritual beliefs of the first inhabitants of Australia. Aboriginal peoples from different parts of Australia have their own names for themselves, such as Koori, Yamaji, Nunga, Murri and Yolgnu. These names are specific to various regions and are only used when referring specifically to that region. Outside of Australia, the term 'aboriginal' is also used as a synonym for 'indigenous'.

Aboriginal and Torres Strait Islander culture is said to be one of the oldest cultures in the world, dating back more than 40,000 years. There have been many debates regarding the number of Aboriginal and Torres Strait Islander peoples and the number of language groups prior to colonisation. The population estimate is dependent on the text source and varies from 300,000 to more than a million, with the number of language groups reported as between 200 and 250.

As tribal peoples, the tangata whenua or Indigenous peoples of New Zealand identify themselves by the names of their hapu (sub-tribe) and iwi (tribe). Renaming was an early process of colonisation and the adjective Maori, meaning ordinary or normal, was used as a noun to 'reidentify' them as one homogenous group (Smith

1999). As it is now universally known, and for the purposes of this chapter, the term Maori is used to refer to the Indigenous peoples of New Zealand.

Maori, Aboriginal and Torres Strait Islander peoples belong to an international network of Indigenous communities who are unified in a collective struggle for their rights as first peoples. These rights are derived from their status as descendants of the original occupants of the lands and territories they now inhabit with others. Those others include the colonisers who have become the majority and migrant or ethnic minorities who came later. In the current fervour to promote 'multiculturalism', it is important to distinguish between Indigenous peoples and ethnic minorities (Maaka & Fleras 2005). Indigenous peoples occupy a unique political space and should not be 'redefined' as ethnic minorities in their own countries. The differences lie in the historical relationship that exists between the Indigenous peoples and the colonising power (the Crown), and their status does not depend on numbers in the population (Jackson, cited in Robson & Reid 2001).

Definition of health and wellbeing

For Aboriginal and Torres Strait Islander peoples and Maori, health is conceptualised differently from those of their governments' policies which reflect the World Health Organization's principles for health and wellbeing[2] (1986). The following statement from the National Aboriginal Health Working Party (1989) provides insight into Australian Indigenous health concepts:

> 'Aboriginal health is not just the physical well being of an individual but is the social, emotional and cultural well being of the whole community in which each individual is to achieve their full potential thereby bringing about the total well being of their community. It is a whole-of-life view and includes the cyclical concept of life-death-life.'

See Box 3.1, which presents an example of the interrelatedness of the child, wellbeing and community.

These views are consistent with Maori health concepts. Mason Durie's Whare Tapa Wha model is a contemporary framework that draws key elements from Maori philosophy to depict health as four dimensional (Durie 1998). Using the walls of a house to symbolise health, these dimensions are named wairua (spirituality), hinengaro (mental wellbeing), whanau (family) and tinana (physical wellbeing). Put simply, health is dependent on the harmony and stability between and within all four dimensions.

History of colonisation and its contemporary effects on Indigenous families

All over the world, colonisation has followed a pattern of cultural destruction, dispossession of people from their land and natural resources, political disempowerment, depopulation and displacement of intellectual traditions (Durie 2005,

2 See Chapter 2 for health promotion principles informing national healthcare policy in Australia and New Zealand.

Box 3.1 Collectivism and Aboriginal childrearing

It is interesting to consider the traditional values of collectivism invested in childrearing practices among Australian Aboriginal peoples, while at the same time being careful to neither stereotype nor homogenise. The literature available around contemporary childrearing practices in Aboriginal Australian families is limited. However, traditional Aboriginal childrearing practices, still influencing Aboriginal families living in remote and many urban parts of Australia, provide some insight into collectivism in childrearing.

The Aboriginal perspective on childrearing is based on a collectivist view of family and social life that sees responsibility for the rearing of children invested in many people. According to this view, children come to trust in the capacity and commitment of a multitude of people to care for them and nurture them through childhood and into adulthood (Howard 2006). A collectivist society depends on their relationships and obligations to significant others. Collectivists describe themselves by referring to the groups they belong to, the land which they are from, and not their individual rewards or results (Howard 2006).

Traditionally, Aboriginal children are seen as self-reliant and are encouraged to regulate their own behaviour and development (Kearins 1984, 2000). In traditional family function, children help care for younger children and assist with household tasks from an early age (Kearins 2000). Independence in learning is highly regarded and developmental skills and behaviour are determined by the child (Kearins 1984). Traditionally, Aboriginal children are raised in an environment that is not verbally directed, nor are they required to stay in close proximity to their carers and are hence relatively free to explore their world. Observational or visual channels are thus important in the learning style.

Aboriginal infants are viewed as autonomous individuals capable of indicating their own needs. It is the signals provided by the infant that will determine a response such as feeding and the need for comfort (Brown 2000). These learning pathways are possible in a collective environment, and contrast with the individualised, regulated and isolated environment of some western childrearing models.

Maaka & Fleras 2005). Following European settlement, Indigenous populations in both Australia and New Zealand rapidly declined as a direct result of conflict and the introduction of European diseases that they had no defences against. The firmly held belief of the European settlers that Indigenous peoples were inferior led to laws that denied them appropriate citizenship (Eckermann et al. 2006). The social and cultural organisations of Indigenous groups were undermined and their spiritual belief systems challenged by both western secular and religious ideas and organisations.

Australia

In Australia, the declaration of European settlers in 1778 that Australia was an empty land, 'terra nullius', had far-reaching consequences that reside today in contemporary Australian society. In 1992, in the historic Mabo decision, the High Court of Australia overturned the ruling of terra nullius, and this paved the way for more appropriate recognition of Aboriginal sovereignty (Bessarah 2000). Aboriginal and Torres Strait Islander peoples traditionally had strong connections between family, culture and the land. The effects of non-Indigenous policies have weakened those links, which in turn has had a major impact on the health of many of these people (Mathews 1998, 2004).

Aboriginal and Torres Strait Islander peoples suffered under various state governments' so-called 'protectionist' policies, such as the Aborigines Protection Act (1869, Victoria), Aborigines Act (1905, Western Australia), and the Aborigines Protection Act (1909, New South Wales). The protection (segregation) policy did not achieve its aims and was replaced by policies of assimilation (1950s–60s). The consequence of both the 'protection' and 'assimilation' policies was that many thousands of Aboriginal children were removed from their parents (Broome 2002). These children are known as the 'Stolen Generation' and a national inquiry into the separation of Aboriginal and Torres Strait Islander children is documented in the 'Bringing them home' report (Human Rights and Equal Opportunity Commission 1997).

The next policy shift was integration (1967–72), encouraging Aboriginal peoples to adopt European ways and abandon their culture (Human Rights and Equal Opportunity Commission 1997). The people of Australia voted in a referendum in 1967 to remove two discriminatory clauses in the 1901 constitution. This resulted in governments being prohibited from passing special laws relating to Aboriginal peoples. Aboriginal peoples were also to be recognised as Australian citizens and be included in the census.

New Zealand

By the time New Zealand was being colonised, Britain had started to acknowledge the harm being brought to Indigenous peoples in territories it had colonised. Unlike Australia, Maori were offered a treaty, and in 1840 the Treaty of Waitangi was signed by Maori and the British Crown. While it is seen as the 'founding document' of New Zealand, it remains the subject of ongoing political and public debate (Durie 1998, Orange 2004, Reid & Cram 2005, Walker 2004).

As an agreement between two parties, the Treaty articulated a relationship between Maori and the Crown and, through good governance promised by the British, Maori would be protected from the detrimental effects of colonisation. The Treaty was written in Maori and English and, according to the Maori text, Maori would retain their lands and natural resources and the right to exercise authority over them (self-determination or tino rangatiratanga) (Durie 1998). Guarantees were also made to Maori in relation to equity and citizenship, ensuring they would have equal access to the benefits of a new society (Reid & Cram 2005).

Debate centres on questions of British intent and motivation for a Treaty and differing perceptions of whether Maori sovereignty was ceded or not. These questions are fuelled by inconsistencies between the Maori and English texts and disagreement about which text is the 'right' one. In reality, and regardless of which text is recognised, the promises in neither text have been fulfilled. Present-day inequalities between Maori and other New Zealanders in social, economic and health status do not reflect good governance or the equity and equal access to the benefits of society promised in the Treaty. Needless to say, nor did Maori retain their land and natural resources, let alone the right to exercise authority over them.

History shows that following the signing of the Treaty of Waitangi, the settler government was quickly established without the Treaty partner, and through mainly legislative process Maori were effectively dispossessed of their land and their sovereignty (Durie 1998, Orange 2004, Walker 2004). Like Australia, assimilation was a key agenda item and, well into the 1960s, policies including urbanisation and other acts of assimilation in New Zealand saw the loss of Maori language, culture, tribal unity and identity—all critical determinants in the health of Indigenous peoples.

Effects on contemporary families

The emergence of Indigenous peoples as a social movement has led to international acknowledgment of the historic and lingering impacts of colonisation on Indigenous communities throughout the world (Sissons 2005, Smith 1999). To appreciate the impact of land loss on the health of Indigenous peoples, it is necessary to understand their relationship with the natural environment. Apart from the universal value of land as an economic base and place to live, for Indigenous peoples the land is the foundation of social unity, cultural identity and the source of spiritual sustenance (Durie 1998, National Aboriginal Health Working Party 1989).

It should need no explanation therefore that when people are dispossessed of their cultural, spiritual, social and economic base, their cultural, spiritual, social and economic wellbeing will suffer—for generations. The present circumstances faced by Indigenous peoples are inextricably linked to the past.

Racism

Given the discussion of historical events and influences on contemporary Indigenous peoples and their health, and before examining more specific health issues, it is necessary to talk about racism. Racism refers to the belief that groups of people are based on genetic similarities rather than on social agreements between people. Racism, like sexism and classism, is about power. 'It is the approach by which one dominant racial group has, and maintains power over another racial group and subordinates it' (Smith 2004).

Most of us would declare ourselves 'non-racist' and would find it difficult to accept that racism continues to be a significant and widespread problem. However, although overt racism has become increasingly socially unacceptable, racism still exists. As Mellor et al. (2001) contend, subtle racism occurs in the context of everyday living, such as shopping, using public transport and eating in restaurants—and, importantly, accessing mainstream services, be it health, welfare, education or the justice system.

Understanding our own prejudices and taking responsibility for how these feelings can affect service delivery is one of the most significant things we can do to improve services for individuals and groups who are marginalised by the system. Most of us do not intend to be racist in our attitudes, but every time we assign a negative feeling towards someone based on their culture, language, behaviour or beliefs, this is racism. It usually happens because we have a different cultural viewpoint from the person to whom we are offering services. These different values and beliefs result in us making assumptions to predict behaviours in individuals or groups who are different from ourselves and can lead us to stereotype or generalise. A stereotype and a generalisation may appear similar, but they function very differently.

A 'generalisation' is a beginning point. It indicates common trends, but further information is needed to ascertain whether the statement is appropriate to a particular individual (Galanti 1991). A 'stereotype' is an endpoint. No attempt is made to learn whether the individual in question fits the statement (Galanti 1991). Stereotyping does not allow for individual differences within cultures and commonly victimises groups by blaming their cultures for perceived and negatively valued practices. In Box 3.2, you will find a reflective exercise that encourages you to challenge the stereotypes.

Box 3.2 Critical questions and reflections: challenging the stereotypes

An Aboriginal health worker (AHW) has been asked to present a workshop to student midwives in a local hospital. To allow sufficient time to set up the room, the AHW arrives 15 minutes prior to the scheduled starting time. The AHW is shy; she sits and waits for the students to arrive. As the students arrive, several of them start a conversation making comments such as 'typical Aboriginal person, always late'; 'I don't know why we have to be here anyway'; 'If they didn't drink, smoke and take drugs so much they would be just the same as everyone else'. The AHW who has fair skin then stands up and says, 'I am the AHW who will be presenting to you today and I was here 15 minutes before you arrived.'

1. What were the preconceived judgments made by the midwives regarding Indigenous peoples?
2. How difficult do you think it may have been for the AHW to continue presenting the workshop given the attitudes of a number of the participants?

An important contributory factor to the poor health status of Aboriginal and Torres Strait Islander peoples and Maori is institutional racism. Institutional racism has been defined as:

> '. . . the ways in which racist beliefs or values have been built into the operation of social institutions in such a way as to discriminate against, control and oppress various minority groups' (Henry et al. 2004).

A number of examples of institutional racism for Aboriginal and Torres Strait Islander peoples are provided below:

» *Funding inequity*: overall funding of Aboriginal healthcare is not commensurate with extra need.

» *Different performance criteria for black and white*: for example, in Perth, Derbarl Yerrigan Aboriginal Medical Service funding was cut when an 'overspend' arose because of success in attracting clients. At the same time, the teaching hospitals' overspend was 120 times greater than that at Derbarl Yerrigan. The teaching hospitals were given an extra $100 million to cover their overspend.

» *'Body part' funding*: separate streams of money are provided for conditions such as diabetes and heart disease for a health service which is intended to be holistic. For example, there are 26 funding streams (and hence 26 separate accounts and 26 demands for accountability) for the Danila Dilba Aboriginal Medical Service in Darwin.

» *Differences in treatment regimens*: Aboriginal peoples in Western Australia born in the 1940s received low-cost nursing care; in contrast, a white cohort of the same age received higher cost technological care.

» *Inequitable Medicare funding of primary healthcare* (Medicare Benefits Schedule plus Pharmaceutical Benefits Scheme): in Katjungka (a remote Aboriginal community), it is $80 per head per year; in Double Bay (an affluent Sydney suburb), it is $900 per head per year.

» *Cultural barriers to Aboriginal use of healthcare services*: there is inadequate funding to reduce these barriers (such as language barriers and lack of recognition of different constructs of health) for Aboriginal peoples (Henry et al. 2004).

To counter overt and covert racism within the Australian health system, a number of principles have been prepared for the *Cultural respect framework for Aboriginal and Torres Strait Islander health 2004–09* (Australian Health Ministers' Advisory Council 2004 pp. 8–9). They include:

» a holistic approach
» health sector responsibility
» community control of primary healthcare services
» working together
» localised decision making
» promoting good health
» building the capacity of health services and communities, and
» accountability for health outcomes.

Determinants of health, and current health status

The relationships between health and social factors including housing, employment, poverty and education have been well documented (Marmot 1998) and it is well established that the health and welfare indicators for Aboriginal and Torres Strait Islander peoples and Maori remain consistently worse than non-Indigenous groups. The relationship between disadvantage and poor health is complex, but the major influences include low educational achievement, low incomes, low employment rates, inadequate housing and transport, exposure to pollutants, poor access to health services and reduced access to healthy foods (Richardson & Prior 2005).

For Indigenous peoples in Australia and New Zealand, the residual effects of land alienation, asset loss and social destruction explain why Maori, Aboriginal and Torres Strait Islander peoples are disproportionately represented in lower socioeconomic strata (Ministry of Health New Zealand 2006). See Chapter 1 for a discussion of social gradient and risks and protective factors for children's health. Table 3.1 offers a summary of the latest demographic data available.

Table 3.1 Demographic data on Indigenous peoples

Indicator	New Zealand	Australia
Population	Total: 4,178,658 Maori: 565,329 (14.6%)	Total: 20 million Aboriginal and Torres Strait Islander: 492,000 (2.4%)
Postschool qualifications	Total: 40% Maori: 30%	Total: 57% Aboriginal and Torres Strait Islander: 32%
Unemployment	Total: 5.1% Maori: 11%	Total: 4.6% Aboriginal and Torres Strait Islander: 13%*
Median income	Total: $24,000 Maori: $20,900	Total: $34,700 Aboriginal and Torres Strait Islander: $20,400
Median age	Total: 35.5 years Maori: 22.7 years	Total: 36 years Aboriginal and Torres Strait Islander: 21 years

* Excludes Community Development Employment Program (Work for the Dole) participants.

Source: Statistics New Zealand census (2006), Ministry of Health New Zealand (n.d.) and Australian Bureau of Statistics (2005).

Maori health

A review of government reports, research and statistical data (Ministry of Health New Zealand 2006, 2005, 2003) illustrates 'systematic disparities in health outcomes, in the determinants of health, in health system responsiveness and in the health workforce' (Reid & Robson 2006). A snapshot of Maori health issues highlights the following disparities: a greater number of low birth weight newborns and greater mortality in the first 5 years of life; the Sudden Infant Death Syndrome rate is four times higher than for non-Maori; children and adolescents have a higher risk of both accidental and non-accidental injury; and rates of youth suicide are increasing, along with mental illness, drug and alcohol abuse, and injury and death from road traffic accidents and violence.

Maori children and young people also have a higher incidence than non-Maori in a range of infectious illnesses, such as pneumonia, tuberculosis, rheumatic fever and, more recently, meningococcal disease. In adulthood, Maori have a higher risk of cancers, cardiovascular disease and diabetes. Maori therefore bear a disproportionate burden of risk, morbidity, disability and mortality in almost every major disease category with the exception of melanoma, which is 'the only area of health in which Maori don't fare worse' (Blakely et al. 2005). Box 3.3 provides a critique of the representation of health embedded in western epidemiological data.

Aboriginal and Torres Strait Islander health

In Australia, Aboriginal and Torres Strait Islander peoples can expect to live 20 years less than non-Indigenous people (Australian Bureau of Statistics 2005). Aboriginal babies are twice as likely to die in the perinatal period and three times more likely to die in infancy (Australian Institute of Health and Welfare 2005). Meningococcal infections are six times higher in the non-Aboriginal and Torres Strait Island population (Olesch & Knight 1999). Rates for Sudden Infant Death Syndrome are eight times higher.

Box 3.3 Critical reflections: explaining ethnic inequalities in health

Although Maori may view access to their language, lands and cultural identity as important indicators of health and wellbeing, they do not discard the standard measures of life expectancy, mortality and morbidity data. There is a concern, however, that data highlighting ethnic disparities focuses on Maori as the 'problem' and that they are somehow deficient and to blame for their poor health.

This 'deficit thinking' fails to consider the possibility that the real deficiencies lie elsewhere. Recent discourse on differential access for Maori to the determinants of health (e.g. income, education and housing, access to healthcare and treatment and quality of care received) has exposed institutional racism and highlighted deficiencies in systems, policies and practices that fail to recognise or respond to Maori needs (Jones 2000, Reid et al. 2000).

From an Indigenous point of view, how data are framed and analysed is critical in determining appropriate responses to improve health services and health outcomes.

Morbidity data indicate that chronic disease (including respiratory disease, cardiovascular disease, renal disease and diabetes) remains the highest causative factor in the morbidity and mortality of Aboriginal and Torres Strait Islander peoples. For children, morbidity statistics indicate that, in 2003–04, Indigenous infants were more likely to be hospitalised than other infants, while Indigenous and other children aged 1–14 years were hospitalised at similar rates.

The prevalence of infections among Aboriginal and Torres Strait Islander children is higher than in non-Aboriginal children in almost every aspect. This is largely due to the higher rates of overcrowding and poverty found in these communities. Ear, skin, respiratory and gastrointestinal systems are all affected. Ear disease, for instance, is endemic in many Aboriginal populations who suffer up to 10 times the rate of otitis media, including chronic suppurative otitis media and consequent hearing loss (Commonwealth of Australia 2001). Hospital admissions for Aboriginal and Torres Strait Islander infants for skin, respiratory system, infectious and parasitic diseases are around three times the rate for other infants (Australian Bureau of Statistics 2005).

The ongoing poor health status of Aboriginal and Torres Strait Islander peoples can be directly attributed to their low social gradient, an ongoing impact of colonisation. Ring and Brown (2002) argue that while there have been strategies and programs to improve access to health services, more needs to be done. It could be argued that the development of additional strategies is wasting resources that should be spent on implementing strategies such as the National Aboriginal Health Strategy (National Aboriginal Health Working Party 1989) that have never been totally implemented (Ring & Brown 2002).

The role of nursing in reducing inequalities

As a nurse or midwife, the extent of disparities in health, and individual capacity to address them, may be overwhelming. However, significant improvements in services can be achieved through individual recognition of:

» the health inequalities that exist and why
» the way continuing with 'doing health business as usual' maintains or increases health inequalities
» how each individual can contribute to change, and
» how each individual can initiate change.

As they represent the largest group of health professionals in health settings, nurses and midwives form a powerful group. Improving access to health services and the quality of health service delivery is within the scope of nursing and midwifery practice and can be a key strategy in reducing inequalities. One means of improving access is in the application of a concept that requires nurses and midwives to analyse the power they hold as individual practitioners and as a collective group.

The idea of cultural safety was conceived by Maori in relation to their concerns about Maori health status and their experiences of culturally inappropriate health services (Ramsden 2002). As a concept it was introduced into New Zealand nursing education in 1990 and has since gained international interest across a range of disciplines. It is often contrasted with the theory of transcultural nursing, which advocates the need to study cultural practices and ideas of population groups in order to provide appropriate nursing care. The significant difference between the two approaches is that cultural safety requires nurses to look at their own cultural practices and ideas, and the impact these may have on clients for whom they are caring (Ramsden & O'Brien 2000).

Cultural safety and Maori

Cultural safety was initiated by Maori about Maori concerns, but since its inception it has undergone a 'metamorphosis' to the point where the concept now relates to all persons. The Nursing Council of New Zealand (2005) defines cultural safety as the effective nursing practice of a person or family from another culture, and that it is determined by that person or family. Culture however extends beyond ethnicity to include age or generation, gender, sexual orientation, occupation and socioeconomic status, migrant experience, religious or spiritual belief, and disability. 'Unsafe cultural practice comprises any action which diminishes, demeans or disempowers the cultural identity and wellbeing of an individual' (p. 4). Unsafe cultural practice is therefore a significant barrier to health service for many people. The dominance of western health policy and services compounds the likelihood of unsafe practice.

Although the theory of cultural safety is no longer specific to Maori, the Nursing Council of New Zealand states that nurses have a social mandate to improve health outcomes for Maori and make explicit their expectations, in *Guidelines for cultural safety: the Treaty of Waitangi and Maori health in nursing practice and education*. For example:

> 'The purpose of cultural safety in nursing education extends beyond the descriptions of practices, beliefs and values of ethnic groups. Confining learning to rituals, customs and practices of a group assumes that by learning about one aspect gives insight into the complexity of human behaviours and social realities. This assumption that cultures are simplistic in nature can lead to a checklist approach by service providers, which negates diversity and individual consideration' (p. 4).

In regard to Indigenous peoples, assumptions cannot be made about cultural identity. As an example, in a midwifery context the spiritual significance for Maori of the whenua (placenta) is recognised and it is common practice now following the birth to offer it to the whanau (family) for burial. This practice is a positive response to the needs of Maori in health service delivery and bodes well for the possibility of future changes. However, for those Maori who have been removed from their cultural information, being offered the whenua could be offensive and even disturbing. The complexity of culturally safe practice becomes abundantly clear in this example and the recent development of Tikanga Best Practice policies by District Health Boards aims to further enhance the provision of culturally safe health service to Maori. These policies take into account diversity among Maori, but reflect widely accepted Maori belief systems and practices related to healthcare.

While it is difficult to measure the effect of cultural safety education and policy in improving Maori health, the success of Maori initiatives in improving access to health services and long-term health gain is more significant (Ministry of Health New Zealand 2002). In the last two decades, the development of Maori health services has provided Maori peoples with more options in terms of health service delivery. These initiatives are still controlled by the Crown, but they reflect in varying degrees the right of Maori to determine their own health outcomes (self-determination).

Culturally safe practice, as a means of improving access to health service and of addressing health inequalities, is simply based on effective communication, analysis of one's own cultural biases and a willingness to neutralise the power imbalance that is inherent in nurse–client relationships. Working in partnership, as discussed in Box 3.4, paves the way for this to happen.

Cultural safety/respect from an Aboriginal and Torres Strait Islander perspective

The *Cultural respect framework for Aboriginal and Torres Strait Islander health 2004–2009* (Australian Health Ministers' Advisory Council 2004) defines cultural respect as 'recognition, protection and continued advancement of the inherent rights, cultures and traditions of Aboriginal and Torres Strait Islander cultures' (p. 7). The framework was developed after extensive consultation to address issues of inequity and cultural safety for Indigenous peoples with the goal being to 'uphold the rights of Aboriginal and Torres Strait Islander peoples to maintain, protect and develop their culture and achieve equitable health outcomes' (p. 7). Furthermore, the framework aims to ensure that cultural respect is embedded into the provision of health service, policies and strategies. It is the responsibility of health service administrators in states and territories to work collaboratively with Aboriginal and Torres Strait Islander peoples to implement the framework at the state and local levels.

The Congress of Aboriginal and Torres Strait Islander Nurses (CATSIN) was established in 1997 as a forum for Aboriginal and Torres Strait Islander nurses. The initial priorities for CATSIN were to improve recruitment and retention of Indigenous nurses and to ensure that CATSIN had input in decision making at all

Box 3.4 Practice highlight: Maori health providers

Turuki Health is a Maori health provider in South Auckland. It provides a range of health and social services, including a team of 'Well Child' nurses, lactation consultants, midwives, disease state management nurses, a general practice, a team of social workers, Kaumatua (Maori elder), as well as traditional Maori health practitioners in the areas of Mirimiri (massage) and Rongoa (Maori medicine). Their approach to health promotion extends far beyond the limitations of health education to include collaboration with other sectors (housing, the local city council, work and income) and participation of community members at governance and other levels.

One of its key services is the Hawaiiki Project, which is a national initiative involving intensive home visiting and follow-up with families who face multiple social and health needs. While the provision of culturally appropriate services is a key factor in improving access, this project aims to address the social and economic barriers that impact on the health of whole families and communities. In partnership with other disciplines, nurses and midwives, both Maori and non-Maori, are playing significant roles in the delivery of these services and are therefore playing significant roles in improving Maori health outcomes.

TAONGA is a facility also in South Auckland that provides secondary school education for teenage mothers and childcare for their infants. The majority of students are Maori and come from the local community. Based at this facility is a Maori nurse whose specialties include Well Child Nursing and Adolescent Health. She collaborates with visiting Plunket nurses, midwives, youth health services, teachers and other community agencies to ensure continuity of care for the students and their babies. Her own role is comprehensive and includes a teaching component covering sexual health, parenting, growth and development, breastfeeding and child protection. She uses the HEADSS assessment tool to identify the needs of the young women and home visiting enhances her ability to support them, their babies and their partners in the context of the wider whanau. The role of this nurse has been critical in the success of students completing their school qualifications and therefore enhancing their health potential in the future.

levels of government. The *Getting em n keeping em* report (2002 p. 50) of the Indigenous Nursing Education Working Group endorsed the Aotearoa model of cultural safety in nursing and midwifery of the Nursing Council of New Zealand.

Cass et al. (2002) promote the development of interpersonal relationships between health service providers and clients as a necessity to improve health outcomes. In their study, Cass et al. advocate the development of strategies for non-Indigenous health service providers to communicate effectively with Indigenous clients and families. While the study was carried out with the Yolngu people (from East Arnhem Land), strategies can be developed and adapted with other Indigenous communities. Strategies could include:

» Indigenous health service providers as cultural advisors
» Indigenous peoples as interpreters
» all staff to complete cultural respect/cultural safety programs
» Indigenous health service providers to be included as part of the multidisciplinary team
» consultation with Indigenous communities, and
» respect for cultural beliefs and practices (Cass et al. 2002).

Box 3.5 provides an example of a strategy and associated team-based service.

Box 3.5 Practice highlight: an Aboriginal maternal and infant health strategy

The New South Wales Aboriginal maternal and infant health strategy (AMIHS) aims to improve the health of Aboriginal women during pregnancy and decrease perinatal morbidity and mortality. This is achieved through the establishment of small teams consisting of a community midwife and Aboriginal health worker (AHW) or a health education officer (AHEO). These teams provide community-based and continuity of care services for Aboriginal women in conjunction with existing medical, midwifery, paediatric and child and family health staff.

The team approach, where an AHW/AHEO and a midwife work together in a primary healthcare model to provide continuity of care, is a major strength of the AMIHS. A number of innovative community development projects have been undertaken as part of the AMIHS. These include art programs, peer education and partnerships with other organisations.

Working in partnership

As already identified, the provision of culturally safe care is reliant on the health provider to recognise the social, cultural and environmental influences on the health of individuals and community groups. Communication in health provider and patient/family relationships was also highlighted above as a critical strategy in improving health outcomes.

Partnership models provide an effective and growing methodology, grounded in strengthening and enabling (see Ch 1 for a discussion of strengths approaches). Partnership models provide an alternative to the long-dominant expert systems model (Giddens 1990) that accompanied biomedical approaches to healthcare. Within this approach the practitioner, as the expert, determines the health needs of clients and offers advice, education and other strategies to address these needs. The expert model assumes domination and control of the health interaction by the professional (Elkan et al. 2000).

This model fails to recognise or respect the centrality of the clients' role in determining their own health. It also fails to address problems that relate to the cultural, social, historical and environmental influences of health and wellbeing. In an area as complex as Aboriginal, Torres Strait Islander and Maori health, the expert model fails to recognise the multiple layers of complexity that influence this population's health and wellbeing.

Working in partnership requires clinicians to transfer the focus of professional attention away from 'problems', 'deficits' and 'weaknesses', and towards the strengths or power of the client or community. This orientates the professional towards developing a collaborative and equal partnership with clients, focusing on building individual, family and community assets (De Jong & Miller 1995). A major premise of the partnership model is that all clients have strengths and capabilities and are more likely to respond to interventions that build on these, rather than identify weaknesses and deficits (Dunst et al. 2002, Darbyshire & Jackson 2004). Partnership models that focus on strengths aim to increase participants' capabilities and feelings of self-worth (Darbyshire & Jackson 2004).

Another important component of the partnership model is that there is an increasing emphasis on the expertise of the client (individual or collective). The assumption is that, with support, clients will discover their own way rather than learning to adopt some 'right way' defined by a clinician (Barnes & Freude-Lagevardi 2003). Family-centred partnership involves professionals and family members working together in 'pursuit of a common goal' and is 'based on shared decision making, shared responsibility, mutual trust and mutual respect' (Dunst 2000).

Developing a client's self-esteem is an important feature of partnership models. Working in a strengths-based or partnership model does not deny the expertise of the professional; it merely identifies the complementary expertise of the client (Davis et al. 2002). A partnership model is particularly important when working with marginalised groups, such as Indigenous peoples who are historically mistrustful of 'experts' or authority figures. An important component of the principle of empowerment, embedded within partnership models, occurs when the professional believes in the client's ability to understand, learn and manage situations (Dunst & Trivette 1996).

Nurses often carry within themselves a heavy sense of their own responsibility that is incompatible with programs that respect clients as experts of their own lives. Shared decision making between professionals and clients is essential, particularly in the area of child health services. All clinicians can examine their own communication style and biases, for our own prejudices and judgments impact greatly on our ability to work in partnership. This awareness is particularly important when working with Indigenous families. If clinicians believe that their clients are unable or unwilling to take control of their own lives, long-term health gains will be difficult to achieve. Working in partnership requires clinicians to assist individuals to develop, secure and use their own resources that will promote or foster a sense of control and self-efficacy (Rodwell 1996). Reflect on these concepts as you undertake the activity in Box 3.6.

Box 3.6 Critical questions and reflections: assessment of an 18-year-old

You have been asked to do a home visit to assess an 18-year-old Aboriginal woman, Jacinta, who is approximately 20 weeks pregnant and has had no antenatal care to date. The occupants of the house are a single mother aged 35 who has diabetes and hypertension, and her four teenage children. Your visit concerns Jacinta, the eldest child. She is 18 and is pregnant with her second baby. The first baby is 15-month-old Tyrone who is not walking, is underweight and has a runny nose and discharging ears. He was born at 32 weeks after a partially abrupted placenta.

Jacinta had a traumatic time with her last baby, especially in the antenatal period where she felt that the midwife and doctors were judgmental and insisted that she must have consumed alcohol and drugs during her pregnancy. She tells you that she does not use drugs or alcohol. She is now 20 weeks pregnant and has not had any antenatal care. She tells you that she has had intermittent vaginal bleeding and she has long periods of nausea and vomiting and generally feeling unwell.

1. How do you imagine this family (in your mind's eye)? What judgments are you likely to make? How easy is it to blame the victim in this instance?
2. How would you go about finding out more about the family's concerns?
3. How might you approach working with this young woman and her family to support her health needs?

Conclusion

The issues for Aboriginal, Torres Strait Islander and Maori children, young people and their families are rooted in the past. However, the means to address them lie in the present. Recognising and accepting these historical influences is imperative for nurses and midwives if they are to develop a critical awareness of how the dominant Australian and New Zealand groups continue to marginalise Indigenous families. Recognising the fundamental right of Indigenous peoples as first peoples to determine their own futures is the broad brushstroke that needs to shape current attitudes. The immediate need is effective health service delivery grounded in cultural safety, where nurses and midwives acknowledge the past and move forward by working in partnership that builds on family and community strengths.

Key points

» Indigenous peoples are distinct from ethnic minorities.
» Colonisation has had a dramatic and long-standing impact on the health of Indigenous peoples in Australia and New Zealand.
» Aboriginal, Torres Strait Islander and Maori conceptualisations of health are all encompassing, inclusive of the individual and collective, physical and metaphysical, and sustain links among people, history and land.
» Continuing social, economic and political processes exist today that contribute to inequalities in health between Indigenous and non-Indigenous peoples.
» Cultural safety and cultural respect are at the heart of reform.
» All nurses and midwives need to practise from a critically self-aware position in order to understand and enact principles of cultural safety.
» Strength-based partnership models of practice are enabling and capacity building. They build respect, esteem and skills.

Useful resources

Australian Bureau of Statistics (ABS) 2005 *The health and welfare of Australia's Aboriginal and Torres Strait Islander peoples*. ABS Cat. No. 4704.0. ABS, Canberra.

Australian Indigenous Health Infonet, a 'one-stop info-shop' for people interested in improving the health of Indigenous Australians: www.healthinfonet.ecu.edu.au/.

Congress of Aboriginal and Torres Strait Islander Nurses (CATSIN): www.indiginet.com.au/catsin/.

Human Rights and Equal Opportunity Commission: www.hreoc.gov.au/Social_Justice/statistics/index.html.

Massey University Maori Studies website. A range of publications on Maori interests are cited, including a bibliography for Mason Durie: http://maori.massey.ac.nz/.

Ministry of Health New Zealand website has a section devoted to Maori health information and publications: www.maorihealth.govt.nz/.

National strategic framework for Aboriginal and Torres Strait Islander peoples' mental health and social and emotional well being 2004–2009, a 5-year plan: www.health.gov.au/internet/wcms/publishing.nsf/Content/health-oatsih-pubs-wellbeing.

Secretariat of National Aboriginal and Islander Child Care Inc. *Footprints. A resource to where we are.* A resource manual for Aboriginal and Torres Strait Islander children services. Available at www.snaicc.asn.au.

Statistics New Zealand: www.stats.gov.tables/population-indicators.htm.

Statistics New Zealand census 2006 *Quickstats about Maori* (revised March 2007). Available at www.stats.govt.nz/census/2006-census-data/quickstats-about-maori/2006.

Tikanga best practice policies. Available internally at Auckland District Health Board and Counties Manukau District Health Board.

Top End Division of General Practitioners, who have produced a resource for health practitioners working in the tropical north, including specific issues with Aboriginal child health: www.tedgp.asn.au/.

Treaty of Waitangi: available on a number of sites. The following provides further historical background to events leading up to and following the Treaty: www.nzhistory.net.nz/category/tid/133.

TUHA-NZ: a treaty understanding of hauora in Aotearoa-New Zealand, Health Promotion Forum, 2002. Available at www.hpforum.org.nz.

References

Australian Bureau of Statistics (ABS) 2005 *The health and welfare of Australia's Aboriginal and Torres Strait Islander peoples*. ABS Cat. No. 4704.0. ABS, Canberra.

Australian Health Ministers' Advisory Council 2004 *Cultural respect framework for Aboriginal and Torres Strait Islander health 2004–2009*. Australian Government, Canberra.

Australian Institute of Health and Welfare (AIHW) Perinatal Statistics Unit 2005 *Australia's mothers and babies 2003, Perinatal Statistics Series No. 16*. Cat. No. PER29, AIHW National Perinatal Statistics Unit, Sydney.

Barnes J, Freude-Lagevardi A 2003 *From pregnancy to early childhood: early interventions to enhance mental health in children and families*. Mental Health Foundation, London.

Bessarah D 2000 Working with Aboriginal families. In W Weeks & M Quinn (eds), *Issues facing Australian families*, 3rd edn. Pearson Education Australia, Sydney.

Blakely T, Tobias M, Robson B et al. 2005 Widening ethnic mortality disparities in New Zealand 1981–1999. *Social Science and Medicine* 61(10):2233–51.

Broome R 2002 *Aboriginal Australians: black responses to white dominance, 1788–2001*. Allen & Unwin, Sydney.

Brown I 2000 The socialisation of the Aboriginal child. In P Dudgeon, D Garvey & H Pickett (eds) *Working with Indigenous Australians: a handbook for psychologists*. Gunada Press, Curtin Indigenous Research Centre, Curtin University of Technology, Perth, pp. 293–305.

Cass A, Lowell A, Christie M et al. 2002 Sharing the true stories: improving communication between Aboriginal patients and healthcare workers. *Medical Journal of Australia* 176(10):466–70.

Commonwealth of Australia 2001 *Systematic review of the management of otitis media in Aboriginal and Torres Strait Islander populations*. National Aboriginal Community Controlled Organisation, Canberra. Available at www.health.gov.au/internet/wcms/Publishing.nsf/Content/health-oatsih-pubs-omp.htm.

Congress of Aboriginal and Torres Strait Islander Nurses (CATSIN) 2006 *Education Statement, Congress for Aboriginal and Torres Strait and Islander Nurses, Sydney.* Available at www.indiginet.com.au/catsin/education.html.

Darbyshire P, Jackson D 2004 Using a strengths approach to understanding resilience and build health capacity in families. *Contemporary Nurse* 18:211–12.

Davis H, Day C, Bidmead C 2002 *Working in partnership with parents: the parent advisor model*. Psychological Corporation Limited, London.

De Jong P, Miller S 1995 How to interview for client strengths. *Social Work* 40:729–37.

Dunst C 2000 Revisiting 'Rethinking early intervention'. *Topics in Early Childhood Special Education* 20:95–104.

Dunst C, Boyd K, Trivette C, Hamby D 2002 Family-oriented program models and professional helpgiving practices. *Family Relations* 51:221–9.

Dunst C, Trivette C 1996 Empowerment, effective helpgiving practices and family-centered care. *Pediatric Nursing* 22:334–43.

Durie M 1998 *Whaiora: Māori health development*, 2nd edn. Oxford University Press, Auckland.

Durie M 2005 Indigenous health reforms: best health outcomes for Maori in New Zealand. Paper presented at the Unleashing Innovation in Health Care Alberta's Symposium on Health, Calgary.

Eckermann A, Dowd T, Chong E et al. 2006 *Binan Goonj: bridging cultures in Aboriginal health*, 2nd edn. Elsevier, Sydney.

Elkan R, Kendrick D, Hewitt M et al. 2000 *The effectiveness of domicillary health visiting: a systematic review of international studies and a selective review of the British literature*. Health Technology Assessment Programme, 4. Available at www.hta.nhsweb.nhs.uk/fullmono/mon413.pdf.

Galanti G 1991 *Caring for patients from different cultures*. University of Pennsylvania Press, Philadelphia.

Giddens A 1990 *The consequences of modernity*. Polity Press, Cambridge.

Henry B, Houston S, Mooney G 2004 Institutional racism in Australian healthcare: a plea for decency. *Medical Journal of Australia* 180:517–20.

Howard D 2006 *Mixed messages: cross-cultural management in Aboriginal community controlled health services*. Phoenix Consultancy, Darwin.

Human Rights and Equal Opportunity Commission (HREOC) (eds) 1997 *Report of the national inquiry into the separation of Aboriginal and Torres Strait Islander children from their families*. Available at www.hreoc.gov.au/pdf/social_justice/bringing_them_home_report.pdf.

Indigenous Nursing Education Working Group 2002 *Getting em n keepin em*. Report to Commonwealth Department of Health and Ageing, Office for Aboriginal and Torres Strait Islander Health. Available at www.health.gov.au/internet/wcms/publishing.nsf/Content/health-oatsih-pubs-gettinem.htm/$FILE/gettinem.pdf. Accessed 3 April 2007.

Jones C 2000 Levels of racism: a theoretical framework and a gardener's tale. *American Journal of Public Health* 90:1212–15.

Kearins J 1984 *Child-rearing practices in Australia: variation with lifestyle*. Education Department of Western Australia, Perth.

Kearins J 2000 Children and cultural difference. In P Dudgeon, D Garvey & H Pickett (eds), *Working with Indigenous Australians: a handbook for psychologists*. Gunada Press, Curtin Indigenous Research Centre, Curtin, Perth.

Kunitz S 2000 Globalization, states, and the health of Indigenous peoples. *American Journal of Public Health* 90:1531–9.

Maaka R, Fleras A 2005 The politics of indigeneity: challenging the state in Canada and Aotearoa New Zealand. University of Otago Press, Dunedin.

Marmot MG 1998 Improvement of social environment to improve health. *Lancet* 351:57–61.

Mathews C 2004 *Healthy children: a guide for child care*, 2nd edn. Elsevier, Sydney.

Mathews J 1998 The Menzies School of Health Research offers a new paradigm of cooperative research. *Medical Journal of Australia* 169:625–9.

Mellor D, Bynon G, Maller J et al. 2001 The perception of racism in ambiguous scenarios. *Journal of Ethnic and Migration Studies* 27:473–88.

Ministry of Health New Zealand (MOH NZ) n.d. Available at www.maorihealth.govt.nz / moh.nsf / index / ma / home.

Ministry of Health New Zealand (MOH NZ) 2002 *He Korowai Oranga: Maori health strategy*. MOH NZ, Wellington. Available at www.moh.govt.nz.

Ministry of Health New Zealand (MOH NZ) 2003 *Decades of disparity: ethnic mortality trends in New Zealand 1980–1999*. MOH NZ, Public Health Intelligence Occasional Bulletin Series. Available at www.moh.govt.nz / PHI / Publications# occasionalbulletin.

Ministry of Health New Zealand (MOH NZ) 2005 *Decades of disparity II: socioeconomic mortality trends in New Zealand 1981–1999*. MOH NZ, Public Health Intelligence Occasional Bulletin Series. Available at www.moh.govt.nz / PHI / Publications#occasionalbulletin.

Ministry of Health New Zealand (MOH NZ) 2006 *Decades of disparity III: ethnic and socio-economic inequalities in mortality, New Zealand 1981–1999*. MOH NZ, Public Health Intelligence Occasional Bulletin Series. Available at www.moh.govt.nz / PHI / Publications#occasionalbulletin.

National Aboriginal Health Working Party 1989 *A national Aboriginal health strategy*. Department of Health and Ageing, Canberra.

New South Wales Health 2004 *Communicating positively: a guide to appropriate Aboriginal terminology*. NSW Department of Health, Sydney. Available at www.health.nsw.gov.au / pubs / 2004 / pdf / aboriginalterminology.pdf0.

Nursing Council of New Zealand 2005 *Guidelines for cultural safety: the Treaty of Waitangi and Maori health in nursing practice and education*. Nursing Council of New Zealand, Wellington. Available at www.nursingcouncil.org.nz.

Olesch C, Knight G 1999 Invasive meningococcal infection in Western Australia. *Journal of Paediatrics and Child Health* 35(1):42–8.

Orange C 2004 *An illustrated history of the Treaty of Waitangi*. Bridget Williams Books, Wellington.

Ramsden I 2002 Cultural safety and nursing education in Aotearoa and Te Waipounamu. Unpublished doctoral thesis, Victoria University, Wellington.

Ramsden I, O'Brien L 2000 Defining cultural safety and transcultural nursing. Kai Tiaka. *Nursing New Zealand* 6(8):4–5.

Reid P, Cram F 2005 Connecting health, people, and country in Aotearoa New Zealand. In K Dew & P Davis (eds), *Health and society in Aotearoa New Zealand*. Oxford University Press, Melbourne, pp. 33–48.

Reid P, Robson B 2006 The state of Maori health. In M Mulholland (ed.), *State of the*

Maori nation: twenty-first-century issues in Aotearoa Reed. Reed Books, Auckland, pp. 17–32.

Reid P, Robson B, Jones C 2000 Disparities in health: common myths and uncommon truths. *Pacific Dialog* 7(1):38–46.

Richardson S, Prior M 2005 Childhood today. In S Richardson & M Prior (eds), *No time to lose: the wellbeing of Australia's children*. Melbourne University Press, Melbourne.

Ring I, Brown N 2002 Indigenous health: chronically inadequate responses to damning statistics [Crisis]. *Medical Journal of Australia* 177(11):629–31.

Robson B, Reid P 2001 *Ethnicity matters: Maori perspectives*. Statistics New Zealand, Wellington.

Rodwell C 1996 An analysis of the concept of empowerment. *Journal of Advanced Nursing* 23:305–13.

Sissons J 2005 *First peoples: indigenous cultures and their futures*. Reaktion Books, London.

Smith J 2004 *Australia's rural and remote health: a social justice perspective*. Tertiary Press, Melbourne.

Smith L 1999 Decolonising methodologies: research and Indigenous peoples. Zed Books, London.

Statistics New Zealand census 2006 *Quickstats about Maori* (revised March 2007). Available at www.stats.govt.nz/census/2006-census-data/quickstats-about-maori/2006.

Walker R 2004 *Ka whawhai tonu matou, struggle without end*, revised edn. Penguin Books, Auckland.

World Health Organization (WHO) 1986 *Ottawa charter for health promotion*. WHO, Geneva. Available at www.who.int/hpr/NPH/docs/ottawa_charter_hp.pdf.

Chapter 4

Practice integrity: advocacy, ethics and legal issues

Jenny Fraser

Learning outcomes

Reading this chapter will help you to:

» explore the role of advocacy in nursing children, young people and their families

» understand the obligation to advocate for children, young people and their families

» consider the relationship between advocacy, ethics and lawful practice

» analyse ethical frameworks for nursing practice

» recognise the relevance of the United Nation's Declaration of the Rights of the Child to nursing practice

» analyse clinical cases to integrate knowledge of advocacy for children, young people and their families, and

» critically analyse the nursing responsibilities and priorities within practice relating to families at risk, children's rights and child protection legislation.

Introduction

Nurses working in paediatric, child and youth health settings operate within a framework that is informed by lawful scope of practice, and ethical standards. This chapter presents a review of the nurse's role as advocate for children, young people and families, and examines this role across the landscape of children's and youth health services.

While nursing shares the role of patient advocate with a number of other health professions, it is notable that nursing has included advocacy in its scope of practice as a fundamental role since the mid-1990s (Mallik & Rafferty 2000). The International Council of Nurses (2006b) lists advocacy as a 'key nursing role', and commitment is expressed through professional codes of conduct set at the domestic level (Australian Nursing and Midwifery Council 2002, New Zealand Nurses Association 1995). The International Council of Nurses (2006a) code of ethics is relevant to nursing practice in both Australia and New Zealand. There are four primary components guiding standards of conduct for nurses:

1. nurses and people
2. nurses and practice
3. nurses and the profession, and
4. nurses and co-workers.

That is, nurses are responsible for acting as advocates for the needs and welfare of patients, for the profession of nursing, and for the interests of colleagues in nursing. Nevertheless, ambiguous interpretations of the concept of patient advocacy continue to pose a number of problems for nurses in practice. Hence, an overview of what advocacy means for nurses working specifically with children, young people and their families is necessary.

Advocacy

The concept of advocacy in nursing has developed over the past three decades from two distinct sources:

1. philosophical writings, and
2. research studies.

Philosophical work and model development was begun in the late 1970s and early 1980s by American writers such as Curtin (1979) and Gadow (1980), and later by Gates (1994) and Mallick (1997a, 1997b, 1998) in the United Kingdom. Models developed from these writings essentially focused on the role of nurses in promoting patient rights and supporting self-care (see O'Connor & Kelly 2005 for a detailed review and critique of these models).

This meant that in assisting patients to exercise their rights to self-determination, nurses were obligated to provide information and support decision making led by patients. The difficulty for nurses was to disentangle dimensions of paternalism and advocacy. O'Connor and Kelly (2005) contend that this led to definitions that simply interpreted patient advocacy as information-giving by nurses and receiving by patients, and that follow-up support by nurses was not incorporated.

A number of research studies have since been conducted to progress the earlier theoretical work by analysing nurses' experiences and perceptions of advocacy (Mallik 1997a, 1997b, 1998, Mallick & Rafferty 2000, O'Connor & Kelly 2005). This body of research has helped to conceptualise advocacy in nursing with some consensus beginning to emerge (Jezewski 1993, Mallik & Rafferty 2000, O'Connor & Kelly 2005).

In their recent study of Irish nurses, O'Connor and Kelly (2005) were able to identify two important elements fundamental to understanding patient advocacy:

1. clinical advocacy, and
2. organisational advocacy.

Specifically, clinical advocacy occurs at a proximal level to the nurse–patient relationship, with nurses acting on behalf of patients regarding healthcare or treatment options, whereas organisational advocacy is more distal. Organisational advocacy involves nurses acting on behalf of patients at a systems level, influencing healthcare options from which they can benefit. Thus, advocacy extends the nurse–patient relationship by integrating the healthcare system. The nurse then mediates or interprets the system as required. This framework attempts to facilitate patient autonomy.

While it may not be possible to offer a precise definition of patient advocacy as it applies to child and youth health nursing practice, it is important to elicit key elements of the concept, including:

» children's rights and healthcare
» decision-making frameworks, and
» ethical decision making and informed consent.

This chapter highlights implications for clinical nursing practice throughout, and then provides more specific reference to child protection legislation influencing nursing practice. Advocacy in the context of therapeutic relationships with children, young people and their families is then considered.

Human rights, child rights and advocacy

The United Nations Declaration of the Rights of the Child (United Nations 1989) sets international standards for protecting the interests and rights of children. The Convention was adopted by the United Nations in 1989 and has been ratified in all but two countries (Somalia and the United States) to date. Australia ratified the convention in 1991, followed by New Zealand in 1993. Despite rights being upheld in legislation, standards and policy, in practice they are not always assured and individual nurses need to advocate for the rights/needs of children, young people and their families at all levels.

Relevant international human rights laws include the child's right to medical treatment located in Article 3 of the Universal Declaration of Human Rights, which provides that 'everyone has a right to life', and Article 12(1) of the United Nation's International Covenant on Economic, Social and Cultural Rights, which recognises 'the right of everyone to the enjoyment of the highest attainable standard of physical and mental health' (cited in Breen 2006 p. 48). Article 19 of the Convention (United Nations 1989) goes further and obligates state parties to intervene to 'protect the child from all forms of physical and mental violence, injury or abuse, neglect or negligent treatment' (cited in Breen 2006 p. 49).

Of particular importance in relation to nursing children and young people is that we accept that individuals have the right to make informed choices about the care they receive. Article 13(1) provides that:

> 'The child shall have the right to freedom of expression; this right shall include the freedom to seek, receive and impart information and ideas of all kinds, regardless of frontiers . . .' (United Nations 1989).

At the same time, advocacy usually means supporting children and young people in the context of their parents' rights and obligations to protect the child. In more recent times, the importance of parental autonomy in child healthcare delivery and decision making has posed the problem of advocacy versus paternalism for nurses practising within a family-centred framework. Advocacy is made more complex when we accept children's rights as paramount. The child's degree of autonomy and capacity to consent to treatment determines their ability to exercise their rights (Breen 2006). As children grow older and develop decision-making skills, their right to consent to treatment and research participation must be respected (Breen 2006).

Practice implications

There is growing support for models of nursing care that are patient-centred. Within paediatric, child and youth health nursing settings, the term 'family-centred care' describes this individualised focus of care. MacKean et al. (2005) argue that family-centred care emerged as best practice in children's health settings from the widespread interest in patient advocacy, citing hospital visiting rights for parents as one outcome of the advocacy movement.

The child (and the nurse) must rely on parents making such treatment and other healthcare decisions based on the child's best interests, as they are recognised as having the authority to act on behalf of the child (Breen 2006). It is therefore important to review models of family-centred care that emphasise training of parents to assume responsibility for care and decision making and move towards truly collaborative relationships between families and nurses.

Advocacy for children, young people and their families extends beyond shifting care responsibility back to families, and requires strategies for the development and maintenance of ongoing collaborative engagements. A key feature of this collaboration is the ability to negotiate plans for care and treatment. The case study in Box 4.1 is designed to illustrate the principles of advocacy in the context of family-centred care. You are encouraged to engage with the related activities.

Box 4.1 Critical questions and reflections: advocacy in family-centred care

A 6-year-old girl, Rebecca, is admitted to the paediatric ward for ongoing surgical treatment to correct congenital talipes. Her mother says that she needs to get back home to care for her other three children and will be back to visit Rebecca in a few days.

1. Reflect on the qualities and skills required to advocate for this family in the practice setting.
2. Consider the advocacy role in relation to the interests and needs of:
   (a) the child
   (b) the parent, and
   (c) the family.

The opportunity for collaborative decision making between the parent and the nurse in this activity at first appears limited. As previously mentioned, collaborative decision making, autonomy and independence are not based on shifting responsibility for care. Rather, consideration is given for the best interests of the family and child.

Decision-making frameworks

Where children cannot consent to participate in treatment or research that will benefit them, either personally or for others, they rely on adults to protect them and to act in their best interests. Children's welfare, meaningful informed consent and respect for patients must therefore be upheld in both treatment and research activities (Diekema & Stapleton 2006). Issues surrounding children and young people's consent to medical treatment will now be examined, followed by those related to children and research.

Using a developmental approach, increasing responsibility is afforded to children in healthcare decisions as they mature. Children in Australia, for example, may assent (voluntarily agree) to treatment or to participate in research before legal autonomy, but it is their parents who must give consent. Box 4.2 provides the guidelines for age-of-majority legislation across Australian jurisdictions.

Box 4.2 Guidelines for age-of-majority legislation in Australia

In most jurisdictions, pursuant to age-of-majority legislation, the age of majority is 18. Beyond that age, people can make their own medical decisions in the same ways as any other adult. In New South Wales and South Australia, the age for making medical decisions is 14 and 16 respectively (*Minors (Property and Contracts) Act 1970* (NSW), section 49). A person who gives medical or dental treatment to a person under the age of 16 is protected from liability if a parent or guardian has consented; a practitioner who performs medical or dental treatment on a person 14 years or older with the consent of that person is similarly protected from liability. In South Australia, under the *Consent to Medical Treatment and Palliative Care Act 1995* (SA), section 6, a person 16 years of age or older may make decisions about their own medical treatment as validly and effectively as an adult.

Adolescence is a particularly challenging developmental stage as young people move towards the autonomy of adulthood. Parental duty to protect the child gives way to the young person's ability to make independent decisions competently (Larcher 2005). Consent for clinical treatment must be adequately informed and freely given by a competent individual. Parents thus have legal power to consent on behalf of the young person if deemed not competent. Difficulty arises when the young person is competent and either refuses treatment or seeks treatment against the wishes of the parents. Interestingly, Breen (2006) argues that, during the past decade, New Zealand's government and judiciary have succeeded in placing children's rights before those of parents. Breen cites a number of cases related to that country's obligations as a State Party to the Convention on the Rights of the Child to uphold Article 6, for example, recognising that 'every child has an inherent right to life in stating that parties should ensure to the maximum extent the survival and development of the child' [1996] NZFLR 670, 671, and using provisions pertaining to 'the right to life in Article 6(1) of the International Covenant on Civil and Political Rights' [198] NZFLR 998, 1000–01, 1003 (cited in Breen 2006 p. 46).

Another fundamental principle in relation to consent to medical treatment is termed 'Gillick competence', which is based on the House of Lords ruling in

Gillick v West Norfolk Area Health Authority 1985 (cited in Breen 2006 p. 54). The Gillick principle holds that some children are legally competent to consent to medical treatment. This ruling only applies to medical treatment that has clear potential for direct benefit to the health of the child. Thus, a 'Gillick assessment' may be used to determine whether a child is 'of sufficient age, maturity and understanding' to consent to medical treatment (Balen et al. 2006 p. 32). In Australia, the law is clear that a child can give legally informed and effective consent to medical treatment using a Gillick assessment, although it is not obligatory. Indeed, it is still argued that Australian law is inadequate in upholding children's rights to medical treatment without parental consent (see, for example, www.hreoc.gov.au/legal/guidelines/submission_michael.htm).

Decision making about the treatment of children and young people is influenced by the values, beliefs and attitudes of the individuals involved. It is important that nurses:

- recognise power inequity in the relationship between parents and the healthcare agency or institution
- enact their role as advocate
- facilitate children's and parents' decision making
- advocate for the child
- assist parents in identifying options consistent with their values, and
- clarify their own values, beliefs and attitudes, and thereby recognise their own biases and potential for influencing parents.

Nevertheless, problems of terminology leave the child at risk, as they are open to interpretation. For example, the concepts of 'best interests' and 'informed consent' are problematic. Moreover, the definitions of child and young person are subject to the various laws in each relevant jurisdiction. Again, the nurse as advocate can play a pivotal role in making sure that risks are reduced and child rights are upheld.

Consider when parents will not give consent for full and complete immunisation for their children as recommended. According to Diekema (2005), there are three important considerations for the healthcare professional:

1. Does this constitute medical neglect and thus reportable neglect?
2. How high is the risk of harm to others?
3. What is the best response?

Diekema (2005 p. 1429) suggests:

- Assess the decision-making framework of the parents.
- Address any misinformation or miscalculation of risk versus benefit.
- Acknowledge risk and the potential for harm, placing it in the context of harm versus benefit.
- Respect the decision (with exception).

Practice implications

The case study in Box 4.3 poses a number of sensitive issues for the school health nurse. On the one hand, the nurse has a responsibility to respect the rights of this child and provide the necessary information and health advice. On the other hand, there is also a duty to uphold the parents' responsibility to protect their child. At the same time, young people have a right to access information and health promoting advice.

Box 4.3 Critical questions and reflections: dealing with sensitive issues

A 15-year-old girl, Angela, arranges an appointment with the school-based nurse. She discloses that she is sexually active and that she is currently not using any form of contraception. Her 15-year-old boyfriend is willing to use condoms, but they do not always use them. Angela implores you not to tell anyone and wants information about how to avoid pregnancy.

1. Reflect on the qualities and skills required of the nurse.
2. What is the role of the nurse as an advocate?

Conflicts between the health system, child and family perspectives on appropriate intervention and treatment may have to be resolved by legal means. This is more clearly understood when the influence of social and cultural context is considered in addition to the cognitive development of children and young people (Hallstrom & Elander 2005). Judgment and decision-making skills develop throughout the early years and are moderated by emotional, cultural and social influences (Jacobs & Klaczynski 2005).

Thus, children and young people's decision-making ability varies within and between communities according to their position within contemporary society. For example, where children are viewed as possessions, the property of their parents and other adults, they are considered vulnerable and dependent. At the other end of the spectrum, children may be viewed as citizens with full rights to express their own opinions and make decisions on their own behalf (Hallstrom & Elander 2005). The school-based nurse (approached by Angela in the case study in Box 4.3) must make clinical decisions based on each of these considerations, the cognitive and emotional development of the child, as well as social and cultural considerations. National and international legislation and conventions designed to protect the rights and interests of children and young people outlined in the previous section must be taken into account.

Ethical decision making and informed consent in research

As previously mentioned, the age at which a child can give informed consent to participate in research and under what conditions they may legally do so relies on individual characteristics, although national regulations exist to protect children in this domain. In Australia, a series of guidelines is available through the National Health and Medical Research Council (2007). Human Research Ethics Committees are charged with the responsibility to ensure that research that does not meet a child or young person's interests does not proceed. The guidelines stress four requisite conditions for the conduct of research with children and young people:

1. the importance of the question
2. that the need for the participation of children/young people is indispensable, as no other source is available to provide answers to the questions

3. the appropriateness of the methodology, and
4. the research is conducted in such a way as to protect their physical, emotional and psychological safety.

The parameters for gaining consent are also stipulated in these guidelines, which state that consent must be gained from:

> '(a) the child or young person whenever he or she has sufficient competence to make this decision; and either
>
> (b) the parents/guardian in all but exceptional circumstances; or
>
> (c) any organisation or person required by law' (p. 26).

The guidelines also stipulate the need for respect for the child and young person's right to refuse to participate.

All the same, the relationship between a child's consent and the consent of parents in social research remains ambiguous in this document. Decision making about children's participation in research continues to be influenced by the values, beliefs and attitudes of individuals (Balen et al. 2006). Shocking medical experiments documented in Nazi concentration camps prompted development of the International Military Tribunal's 10-point code known as the Nuremberg code (Annas & Grodin 1995).

This was the only international code of research ethical standards until 1964 when the *Declaration of Helsinki* was adopted by the World Medical Association Document 17.C (1964, revised 1974, 1983, 1989, 1996, 2000, 2002, 2004). The *Declaration of Helsinki* was established following a powerful history of children's rights abuses in research participation (see Diekema 2006) and has resulted in the adoption of a set of child-specific principles (World Medical Association 2005). The declaration states explicitly that 'permission from the responsible relative replaces that of the subject' (World Medical Association 2005). Children therefore rely on the 'responsible relative' to make decisions on their behalf. At the same time, children must assent to participate. Indeed the policy (World Medical Association 2004) states:

> 'When a subject deemed legally incompetent, such as a minor child, is able to give assent to decisions about participation in research, the investigator must obtain that assent in addition to the consent of the legally authorized representative.'

The requirement for informed consent and provision of an appropriate, usually written, explanation of the study is a critical element. This is where the nurse can act in the role of patient advocate. Everyday plain language must be used without losing the essence of the study's intention and risks (Green et al. 2003). Consideration must be given to parent's literacy capacity. The Australian Bureau of Statistic's report on Australian population literacy levels (1997) provides strong evidence for the need to ensure that parents are well informed if written explanations for consent are relied on. For example, only 17% (2.3 million) of Australians aged 15–74 years were assessed as having good to very good prose literacy skills, and almost half (6.2 million) had 'poor' or 'very poor' skills. Another 35% (4.7 million) of Australians held minimum proficiency, being able to just cope with everyday life needs for literacy. Therefore, information provided to parents for gaining consent must be targeted to the ability of simple or minimum levels of literacy competency (Green et al. 2003).

Useful guidelines and considerations are presented in Box 4.4 for nurses planning to do research with children.

Box 4.4 Practice highlight: tips for writing a human research ethics proposal

- The child must assent to participation according to the World Medical Association (2004) principle.
- The child's assent is given in addition to the consent of the legally authorised representative (usually the parent).
- Parental consent provides consent to approach the child to participate and does not override the child's right to refuse to participate.
- Children as young as 5 years are capable of giving voluntary assent.
- Informed assent means that the child agrees to the conditions of participation.
- All information about the research must be provided in developmentally appropriate terms.
- The child's participation is voluntary and assent is sought away from parental influence.

Child protection and legislation

Within Australian and New Zealand societies the dynamics of the family have changed considerably over recent decades. One such change has been the rising numbers of blended families with step-parents and single-parent families raising children with little and sometimes no extended family support (de Vaus 2004). The rising incidence and changing patterns of illicit drug use is another and extends into the population of women of childbearing age. Escalating use of psycho stimulants in particular, for which we have few treatment options, challenges delivery of health services (Australian Institute of Health and Welfare 2005).

Nurses can find they are in a unique position to support and advocate for children, young people and their families living in such adversity. With that role comes a legal, moral and ethical responsibility that must be clear for the nurse. The prevention of child abuse and neglect (CAN) is a complicated issue involving a multifaceted response from health providers and other relevant services.

The legal duty of nurses to report suspected child abuse and neglect varies across Australian and New Zealand jurisdictions (see Mathews et al. 2006). There are differences in the extent of the duty, the extent of the harm caused to the child that qualifies as reportable, and the type of abuse. Differences occur between jurisdictions on whether it applies to cases of past CAN, perceived likely future CAN, or both. Nurses need to be familiar with the legislation that exists in the particular state or territory in which they work.

For example, Queensland and Victoria impose a condition on the consequences of sexual abuse to make it reportable, while five other jurisdictions do not (Mathews et al. 2006). The broad definition of reportable neglect in New South Wales relies on sound assessment if high rates of unsubstantiated reports are to be avoided. Child abuse and neglect are concepts that are defined by communities with much variation. Similarly, the response of these communities to child abuse and neglect also varies considerably (Mathews et al. 2006). Consider the critical questions and reflections in Box 4.5 to further explore the complex nature of these concepts.

Box 4.5 Critical questions and reflections: personal response to abuse

Parents often compare the school performance of their 16-year-old son Peter to the performance of other boys (and their own), and they tell him he will never amount to anything. They ridicule, criticise and punish him when he does not do well in exams. Peter shows signs of depression and anxiety.

1. If this occurred in your jurisdiction, would you be legally required to report?
2. Do you think that reporting the abuse or neglect is in the child's best interest?
3. Do you think that reporting the abuse or neglect is in the family's best interest?

Clearly, the opportunity to act as patient advocate for children, young people and their families is a privilege. Not only must the nurse be aware of the community standards and legal obligations for reporting, but also as an advocate they must inform and support families to be aware of what is acceptable and what is not. At the same time, it is important to remember that advocacy can, and often does, lead to conflict. When confronted by conflicting commitments and responsibilities, the nurse must make an assessment of risk and act legally and ethically (Mallick 1997a). At the same time, commitment to supporting a family in their actions or decisions for their child may need to be compromised. This is a moral choice, but one that is constrained by legal mandates (e.g. to report suspected child abuse or neglect) and institutional power. The decision to advocate for children, young people and their families can have damaging effects on nurses if risks are taken. Effects include emotional and psychological trauma. Legal penalties may be applied. Consider the legal implications of findings from research presented in Box 4.6.

Box 4.6 Research highlight: reporting of child abuse

In a South Australian study, nurses reported that they had not, in some cases, reported suspected cases of child abuse and neglect despite a legal mandate to do so (Nayda 2002, 2004). Nayda's (2004) research showed that reluctance to report was motivated by concerns for poor outcomes for both the nurse and the family. She also found differences between reporting by paediatric and emergency department nurses, with emergency department nurses more likely to shift responsibility to medical staff, and paediatric nurses more confident in their ability to assess and report suspected cases.

Moreover, serious concerns held by community-based nurses about reporting influenced reporting practice in this study. Nurses experienced tension among their responsibilities. Accountability for supporting high-risk families by a) maintaining therapeutic relationships and b) having concern for the continuing welfare of reported cases was at odds with assuming a role of surveillance.

It is important to contextualise these judgments within lawful scope of practice, and ethical standards. Consider a relationship that is truly collaborative. Parents do not wish to expose their children to harm. At the same time, the nurse practises within a framework that is principled, moral, ethical and legal. Respect for each of these positions within the collaborative and therapeutic relationship assists in taking actions in the best interests of the child and family.

Therapeutic relationships, advocacy and the context of child protection

Therapeutic relationships are a feature of nurse / child / family relationships across the range of services found both in acute care settings for sick children and young people as well as community healthcare settings for well children and young people. Specific characteristics of these relationships and how they differ are detailed in Chapter 5, but for the purpose of this chapter they are referred to more broadly. Nurses are responsible for structuring the relationship so that boundaries remain intact and the advocacy and caring roles are preserved.

Families with particular characteristics face increased challenges in raising their children. The contemporary emphasis on early intervention and prevention programs for such families reflects wider concern that child abuse and neglect are more about parenting capacity, or parental competence and emotional regulation, than individual psychopathology.

The focus is on the parent–child relationship and the way in which the parent responds to behavioural and emotional development of the child. Nurses in clinical practice across the range of healthcare settings play a significant role in this effort.

It is important that the nurse has high levels of knowledge and is alert to and conscious of any emotional reactions, discomfort or feelings that may influence their ability to remain objective and interact in a non-judgmental manner. An awareness of biases, projected opinions and feelings is also important, as it is these subtle cues that a child or parent may pick up on that impact negatively on the therapeutic relationship (Davis et al. 2002).

The nurse's counselling and interpersonal skills are essential to the initiation and maintenance of these relationships (Davis et al. 2002). All forms of neglect and abuse have significant detrimental effects on a child's physical or emotional health, development and wellbeing. Abuse may be one or a combination of the four major types: physical abuse, sexual abuse, psychological / emotional abuse or child neglect. In all forms of abuse, there is almost always an element of emotional abuse. Variations occur due to a variety of risk and protective factors operating within the individual and the environment within which the abuse occurs (Finkelhor & Jones 2006).

Read the case study in Box 4.7 before completing the reader activities related to nurses' legal position, advocacy role and skills required. Whether or not the nurse is required by law to report this as a case of suspected child abuse, there is an ethical and moral obligation to protect Troy from further harm. This would require an extended and ongoing relationship between the nurse and Troy's family. The action to report the abuse to the appropriate authority should not impose on this relationship, but enhance its influence by providing valuable assistance and support not previously available. On the other hand, the results of Nayda's (2004) research indicate that many nurses do not believe that this is a possible outcome and that the family is more likely to be alienated from mainstream services.

Box 4.7 Critical questions and reflections: legal position, advocacy and skills

Troy is a quiet and shy 10-year-old boy. He confides to the school nurse that he is very sad because he accidentally broke his dad's favourite mug. He says his dad told him he was worthless, should never have been born, and was nothing but trouble. When you ask, Troy says that this is how his father always talks to both him and his mother, and that it is okay because his father never really does anything to hurt them.

Legal position

1. In your opinion, do you think that this is a case of child abuse? Why or why not?
2. Is it reportable by law in your jurisdiction? If yes, is it reportable by a registered nurse and to whom does the nurse report?
3. How much harm to the child does there need to be for a report to be made?
4. Do you fear reprisals from reporting suspected or known child abuse? If so, why?
5. Do you fear reprisals from not reporting suspected or known child abuse? If so, why?

Advocacy role

1. Do you think it is in the child's best interests to report child abuse? Why or why not?
2. Do you think it is in the family's best interests to report child abuse? Why or why not?

Skills and competencies

1. What would be your personal strengths as a nurse in this case?
2. What would be your personal limitations as a nurse in this case?

Nurses in a position to develop and maintain productive relationships with families of vulnerable children are often those in a position to make regular home visitations. Opportunities to work closely with families in a sustained way, such as through a home-visitation service, are crucial to assisting families struggling with the demands of parenting. However, it is worth noting that in a recent study of home visitation in the US, home-visiting nurses reported that they had been drawn to working in a home-visiting service for the opportunity to work intensively with vulnerable and high-risk families (Zeanah et al. 2006). However, they were initially unprepared for the intensity and chronicity of their caseloads, citing intimate-partner violence, child abuse, incest and psychopathology as:

» characteristics that interfered with the success of their home-visiting work, and
» requiring mental health nursing skills beyond the base training of home-visiting nurses (Zeanah et al. 2006).

Current initiatives in the suite of home-visiting strategies thus include those targeting specific high-risk family factors such as domestic violence and parental psychopathology (Boris et al. 2006).

If a constructive effort is to be made to assist and support families to establish effective parenting, it is crucial that nurses avoid critical, judgmental or aggressive attitudes towards possible perpetrators. Specific training is required and if the research summarised above continues to demonstrate effective outcomes for children, nurses will be increasingly engaging in more specific home-visiting treatments. While most parents easily engage in the therapeutic relationship, the most vulnerable families tend to be those least likely to access services. Remember that healthcare professionals, and the services they represent, may be perceived as the 'wolf in sheep's clothing', with the single intention to report suspected child abuse or neglect. This can occur especially in families who already feel alienated by mainstream services (Fraser et al. 2000).

Conclusion

This chapter explored the role of advocacy within the scope of nursing children, young people and their families. The tensions between advocacy, ethics and lawful practice were considered within the framework of therapeutic relationships with families and the overall issue of children's and young people's safety. Clinical cases were highlighted to integrate an understanding of advocacy within healthcare practices and nursing responsibilities and priorities relating to families at risk, children's rights and child protection legislation.

Key points

» Advocacy is a key role in nursing children, young people and their families.
» Moral, ethical and legal obligations impact on advocacy for children, young people and their families.
» Frameworks for contemporary nursing practice include concepts of therapeutic relationships, collaboration and family-centred care.

Useful resources

An Bord Altranais (Irish Nursing Board): www.aba.ie.
Australian Equal Rights and Equal Opportunity Commission: www.hreoc.gov.au/.
Australian Institute of Family Studies: www.aifs.gov.au/institute/pubs/diversity/main.html.
Australian Nursing and Midwifery Council: www.anmc.org.au.
International Council of Nurses: www.icn.ch.
National Council of State Boards of Nursing (United States): www.ncsbn.org.
Nursing and Midwifery Council (United Kingdom): www.nmc-uk.org.
United Nations Convention on the Rights of the Child (2001): www.unhchr.ch/pdf/report.pdfANMC. A full list of countries that have ratified the convention is provided.

References

Annas GJ, Grodin MA 1995 *The Nazi doctors and the Nuremberg Code: human rights in human experimentation*. Oxford University Press, New York.

Australian Bureau of Statistics (ABS) 1997 *Aspects of literacy: assessed skill levels, Australia*. Cat. No. 4228.0. ABS, Canberra.

Australian Institute of Heath and Welfare (AIHW) 2005 *National drug strategy household survey—detailed findings*. Cat. No. PHE 66. AIHW, Canberra. Available at www.aihw.gov.au/publications/index.cfm/title/10190.

Australian Nursing and Midwifery Council (ANMC) 2002 *Code of ethics for nurses in Australia*. ANMC, Canberra.

Balen R, Blyth E, Calabretto H et al. 2006 Involving children in health and social research. *Childhood* 13(1):29–48.

Boris N, Larrieu J, Zeanah P et al. 2006 The process and promise of mental health augmentation of nurse home-visiting programs: data from the Louisiana nurse–family partnership. *Infant Mental Health Journal* 27(1):26–40.

Breen C 2006 *Age discrimination and children's rights: ensuring equality and acknowledging difference*. Martinus Nijhoff Publishers, Boston.

Curtin L 1979 The nurse as advocate: a philosophical foundation for nursing. *Advances in Nursing Science* 1(3):1–10.

Davis H, Day C, Bidmead C 2002 *Working in partnership with parents: the parent adviser model*. Psychological Corporation, London.

de Vaus D 2004 *Diversity and change in Australian families: statistical profiles*. Australian Institute of Family Studies, Canberra.

Diekema D 2005 Responding to parental refusals of immunization of children. *Pediatrics* 115(5):1428–31.

Diekema D 2006 Conducting ethical research in pediatrics: a brief historical overview and review of pediatric regulations. *Journal of Pediatrics* 149:3–11.

Diekema D, Stapleton FB 2006 Current controversies in pediatric research ethics: proceedings introduction. *Journal of Pediatrics* 149:1–2.

Finkelhor D, Jones L 2006 Why have child maltreatment and child victimisation declined? *Journal of Social Issues* 62(4):685–715.

Fraser JA, Armstrong KL, Morris J et al. 2000 Home visiting intervention for vulnerable families with newborns: follow-up results of a randomised controlled trial. *Child Abuse and Neglect* 24(11):1399–429.

Gadow S 1980 Existential advocacy: philosophical foundation in nursing. In SF Spicker & S Gadow (eds), *Nursing images of reality*. Springer, New York, pp. 79–101.

Gates B 1994 *Advocacy: a nurses' guide*. Scutari Press, London.

Green JB, Duncan RE, Barnes GL et al. 2003 Putting the 'informed' into 'consent': a matter of plain language. *Journal of Paediatrics and Child Health* 39:700–3.

Hallstrom I, Elander G 2005 Decision making in paediatric care: an overview with reference to nursing care. *Nursing Ethics* 12(3):223–38.

International Council of Nurses (ICN) 2006a *The International Council of Nurses' code of ethics for nurses*. Available at www.icn.ch/icncode.pdf.

International Council of Nurses (ICN) 2006b *The International Council of Nurses' definition of nursing*. Available at www.icn.ch/definition.htm.

Jacobs JE, Klaczynski PA 2005 *The development of judgement and decision making during childhood and adolescence*. Lawrence Erlbaum Associates, New Jersey.

Jezewski MA 1993 Culture brokering as a model for advocacy. *Nursing in Health Care* 14:78–85.

Larcher V 2005 Consent, competence, and confidentiality. In R Viner (ed.), *ABC of adolescence*. Blackwell, Oxford, pp. 5–8.

MacKean GL, Thurston WE, Scott CM 2005 Bridging the divide between families and health professionals' perspectives on family-centred care. *Health Experiences* 8(1):74–85.

Mallik M 1997a Advocacy in nursing—a review of the literature. *Journal of Advanced Nursing* 25:130–8.

Mallik M 1997b Advocacy in nursing—perceptions of practising nurses. *Journal of Clinical Nursing* 6:303–13.

Mallik M 1998 Advocacy in nursing: perceptions and attitudes of the nursing elite in the United Kingdom. *Journal of Advanced Nursing* 28:1001–11.

Mallik M, Rafferty AM 2000 Diffusion of the concept of patient advocacy. *Journal of Nursing Scholarship: An Official Publication of Sigma Theta Tau International Honor Society of Nursing/Sigma Theta Tau* 32(4):399–404.

Mathews B, Walsh K, Fraser JA 2006 Mandatory reporting by nurses of child abuse and neglect. *Journal of Law and Medicine* 13(4):505–17.

Meaux JB, Bell PL 2001 Balancing recruitment and protection: children as research subjects. *Issues in Comprehensive Pediatric Nursing* 24(4):241–51.

National Health and Medical Research Council (NHMRC) 2007 *National statement on ethical conduct in human research*. NHMRC, Canberra.

Nayda R 2002 Influences on registered nurses' decision making in cases of suspected child abuse and neglect. *Child Abuse Review* 11(3):168–78.

Nayda R 2004 Registered nurses' communication about abused children: rules, responsibilities and resistance. *Child Abuse Review* 13(3):188–99.

New Zealand Nurses Association (NZNA) 1995 *Code of ethics*. NZNA, Wellington.

O'Connor T, Kelly B 2005 Bridging the gap: a study of general nurses' perceptions of patient advocacy in Ireland. *Nursing Ethics* 12(5):453–67.

United Nations (UN) 1989 *Convention on the rights of the child*. UN, New York. Available at www.unhchr.ch/pdf/report.pdfANMC. Accessed 14 August 2006.

World Medical Association (WMA) 2004 *Ethical principles for medical research involving human subjects*. Helsinki: 18th World Assembly, 1964. Revised 54th WMA World General Assembly, Tokyo.

World Medical Association (WMA) 2005 *Recommendations guiding medical doctors in biomedical research involving human subjects*. Helsinki: 18th World Assembly, 1964. Revised 52nd WMA World General Assembly, Edinburgh.

Zeanah P, Larrieu J, Boris N 2006 Nurse home visiting: perspectives from nurses. *Infant Mental Health Journal* 27(1):41–54.

Chapter 5

Communication and therapeutic relationships

Judith Rorden

Learning outcomes

Reading this chapter will help you to:

- describe differences in the kinds of relationships nurses have with children, young people and families
- list the characteristics and goals of a therapeutic relationship
- describe why families are the focus of therapeutic relationships in the care of children and young people
- give examples of how communication with children differs according to their age and cognitive development
- discuss the meaning of the phrase 'use of self' as it applies to therapeutic relationships with children, young people and families
- discuss aspects of non-verbal communication that facilitate helping and therapeutic relationships, and
- understand the relationship between communication and assessment, supportive and educational interventions.

Introduction

This chapter begins with a discussion of communication as the basis of a therapeutic relationship. When a child or young person is unwell, the primary therapeutic relationship is most often with both the child and the family. Aspects of communication with families are discussed, along with the effect on communication of the chronologic and cognitive development of the child. The characteristics and goals of a therapeutic relationship are compared with other kinds of helping relationships.

Nurses use both their personal characteristics and their communication skills to develop a therapeutic relationship. The 'use of self' is discussed in terms of the characteristics of empathy, acceptance and genuineness. Both non-verbal and verbal communication skills are explored, along with their place in establishing and maintaining a helping and therapeutic relationship.

Therapeutic relationships with patients and families seek to enable people to build and effectively use their strengths and resources for good health outcomes. The relationship between communication and assessment and intervention practices is explored.

Communication as the basis of therapeutic relationships

Communication is usually defined as the giving and receiving of messages or, perhaps more appropriately, the exchange of meaning. While these very simple definitions are a good starting point, they do not capture the complex nature of the communication that takes place between nurse and patient or family within the context of a therapeutic relationship. For a child or young person who is physically and/or emotionally dependent on their family, healthcare necessarily involves members of that family as well as the patient. In reality, the nurse forms a therapeutic relationship with the family, not with just the patient.

Levels of interaction in nurse–patient and nurse–family relationships

Nurses have many different kinds of relationships with patients and families, ranging from the very superficial to the intensely personal. Interactive communication is central to all of these relationships. One way of distinguishing between them is in terms of the level of interactive involvement (Graber & Mitcham 2004). Quality and quantity are relevant, along with the willingness to reveal something of oneself on the part of both nurse and patient. Stein-Parbury (2005) calls these characteristics mutuality and reciprocity.

One way of distinguishing between levels of complexity in interactive involvement is to look at how the nurse interprets a person's ability and willingness to participate in interaction and how that interpretation guides the nurse's approach. Look at the following examples.

The nurse approaches a recently admitted young child with a smile and a friendly greeting. She recognises that friendly gestures are especially important when working with young children (Berk 2006). Unlike older children and adults who have some expectation of a health professional's goodwill, youngsters who are out of their own environment tend to treat strange adults with suspicion or even fear unless a deliberate attempt is made to dispel negative responses. Although superficial and involving only limited interaction, the nurse's intention in this instance is just to reassure the child that the nurse's care will be given with goodwill and kindly attention.

In the second example, imagine you are the nurse interacting with a family about their young child's chronic asthma. You know that the family has managed the asthma for some time, but that there was a recent acute episode. The mother asks a number of questions about the child's asthma and care for the child. On this basis, you identify a 'clinical relationship' (Stein-Parbury 2005) as appropriate to the situation. The major focus of the communication between you and the mother is on clinical information. You explain procedures, answer questions and assess the mother's understanding about the care of her child. Your intentions are to involve the child and parent in care, keep them informed about medical priorities and decisions, alert them to the reasons for treatment and prepare them to continue care outside the clinical environment.

Therapeutic relationships are often marked by more intense involvement and interaction between patient, family and nurse. They are distinguished by a focus on the feelings as well as the facts affecting the person of concern. Many authors have referred to this as a 'helping' relationship so as to distinguish it from psychotherapy (e.g. Brammer & MacDonald 2003, Ivey & Ivey 2003). Its goals are to enable the person to take appropriate action on their own behalf, enable problem solving and strengthen their resources and those of their family. Therapeutic relationships are appropriate in situations in which people are especially vulnerable to feelings of helplessness or are overwhelmed by circumstance (Stein-Parbury 2005). Examples of such situations are acute health episodes, both physical and mental, diagnoses of life-changing or life-threatening conditions, death of a family member and relationship crises.

In a therapeutic relationship, the nurse deliberately uses their personality, knowledge and skills to establish and maintain communication with patients and families. This deliberate use of skills and personal characteristics by the nurse to further communication is referred to as 'use of self' and was given particular attention by nursing theorists such as Peplau and Travelbee (McEwan & Wills 2002).

The importance of the use of self in therapeutic communication is sometimes overlooked in the current emphasis on biomedical science and economic rationalism (Jackson & Borbasi 2000). Indeed, one Australian study (Gardner et al. 2001) showed that both patients and nurses shared the perception that nurses' technological skills were the most important aspect of nursing care. Yet it is clear that, in all areas of nursing, nurse–patient and nurse–family relationships are central to meeting the needs of the whole person. It is an area of professional practice that can contribute substantially to nurses' personal satisfaction with nursing. It warrants attention as an important area of practice development throughout a nurse's career.

Nurse–family communication

The health and wellbeing of the family unit and the ability of family members to communicate with one another and with the larger community are central to the health of the child or young person and, indeed, to all family members and to broader society (Australian Institute of Health and Welfare 2005). Family functioning can be understood as a system with component parts that are separate but interdependent. That system is capable of growth and development, and is able to achieve more as a unit than could its individual members (DeFrain 1999). (See Ch 1 for further discussion of family.) A nurse's understanding of the composition and functioning of a child's or young person's family allows the nurse to help family members mobilise resources and identify strengths. Every family is unique in the strength of its bonds and its boundaries, and these are formed in complex interactions of cultural and individual dynamics (Smith 2002).

One factor that families share, whatever their shape or size, is that the illness or injury of one member is a major stress if not a crisis for the entire family. This is particularly true when a child or young person is involved. Sometimes, families expand their boundaries in times of crisis. Family members who are not usually highly involved come to offer help, which at times is strengthening, but, in some situations, may contribute inadvertently to the family's stress level. Information about how a family is experiencing their present circumstances, who is involved and what level of support is being offered is important to nurses for developing helpful relationships with family members.

The purposes for establishing and maintaining therapeutic relationships with families parallel those of working in this way with individuals. By helping families identify both the facts and feelings of their situation, nurses help them grow and develop. A nurse's communicative approach can enable a family to make decisions and take positive action towards better physical and mental health for their members.

Age-specific strategies for communicating with children and youth

Whether in hospital, clinic or community, the importance of nurses' skill in communicating with children and young people cannot be overestimated. The quality of that communication not only allows the child or young person to express needs, but also encourages the trust of family members. Observing that a child trusts a nurse and hearing communication between nurse and child, a parent is likely to also feel that the nurse is trustworthy (Shepherd 2001).

The nature of a nurse's relationship and communication with a child or young person will depend on their age, cognitive ability and the willingness to interact. The nurse adjusts verbal and non-verbal communication to their needs and abilities, just as medication doses are adjusted to a child's weight (Stein-Parbury 2005). Children respond to the same kinds of qualities in the nurse as do young people and adults. The nurse encourages their trust by demonstrating warmth and respect. One way in which respect is demonstrated is by not pressuring a child to form a relationship, but rather to offer concern and communication, and allow the child to advance the relationship as trust develops.

In the next paragraphs, the cognitive and communicative developmental stages of children will be revised. Examples of behaviours that engender positive relationships will be provided. Chronological age will be used as an indicator of typical cognitive and psychosocial development. In actuality, the stages tend to blend and overlap for any one unique individual (Bastable 2006). The work of Piaget (1951) and Erikson (1963) provides the framework for discussing interaction with children and young people. See Table 10.1 in Chapter 10 for a summary of child and adolescent psychosocial developmental stages and tasks.

Infancy (0–12 months)

A time of complete dependency, this is the period in which an infant forms attachments with others and begins to explore the social and physical world. Erikson identified the major psychosocial task of this period as resolving trust versus mistrust. If the infant's needs for food, comfort and security are met, trust develops. Without these protective resources, the world may be perceived as an uncertain place.

Both parents and infants are vulnerable during this period. A nurse's communication with the child is related to meeting basic needs and expressing warmth and security. Consistency is important. A nurse has an opportunity during this period of forging an alliance with parents in giving the best possible care to the child. If the infant is ill or has a disability, it is important that parents be helped to express and explore their emotion and reactions, and search for ways to actively support their child that are appropriate to the situation. Because of their feelings of vulnerability, parents can feel challenged by carers who seem to be replacing them in a parental role (Shephard 2001). A therapeutic relationship between nurse and parents aimed at reassurance and partnership with the nurse will reduce anxiety and enable parents to develop skills and take an active role in care. See Chapter 7 for further discussion of early parenting and parenting support.

Toddlers (1–3 years)

Piaget identifies these early years as a 'sensorimotor' period in which the young child learns through the senses. Toddlers learn about their world by physically exploring it, tasting it and listening to it. Language development is extremely rapid (Berk 2006). Erikson called this a period in which autonomy versus shame can be resolved. Children who are allowed to explore and satisfy their curiosity develop a growing sense of self-control and autonomy. Those who are unable to do this because of parental controls, environment or physical disability can become uncertain and fearful (McDevitt & Ormrod 2002).

Around the age of 2 years, the child develops 'object permanence'—that is, where the child develops the ability to understand that just because a person or object is out of sight does not automatically mean that it has ceased to exist. Prior to the development of this concept, the departure of a parent leads to feelings of abandonment. Thus nurse–child communication is focused on reassurance (Bastable 2006). Children of this age are easily distracted and can replace fearfulness with interest in a new toy or activity.

Movement is a major form of communication for toddlers. The actions of enthusiasm and acceptance are easy to interpret, but other kinds of non-verbal communication are not always so. For example, a young child in pain may lie very still rather than cry. This behaviour can be open to misinterpretation by an adult who may believe the child is comfortable.

While language development is very rapid in these years, children understand a great deal more than they can express. Simple explanations and repetition are valuable communication tools. Some parents find that teaching their child sign language for important concepts like 'more' and 'I love you' significantly increases the child's interaction with others.

A nurse's interest in the toddler's preferences, favourite toys and usual routine is a useful way to establish communication with the family and encourage trust. A therapeutic relationship will help a parent realise their strengths and cope with the intense emotions generated by a toddler's illness or injury.

Preschool (4–5 years)

Piaget called the preschool years 'pre-operational' and Erikson identified the psychosocial task as being 'initiative versus guilt'. If children have accomplished previous psychosocial tasks positively, they will have developed a sense of purpose and be able to independently plan and undertake activities. If they are prevented from developing initiative, they will experience a sense of guilt about expressing their needs and desires (McDevitt & Ormrod 2002).

By the time children have reached the preschool years, their fine muscle control allows them to do many tasks of daily living, although they still require adult supervision. Their world expands beyond the immediate family and they learn through play.

Communicating with preschool children still requires simple, very concrete language, but they are better able to remember and categorise speech-based information (Berk 2006). They can be quite concerned about being ill or injured, so adults need to use positive rather than threatening terms to describe events. For example, 'cut' and 'dressing' might be frightening or confusing, while 'fixing' or 'bandaids' are known ideas and more easily accepted (Bastable 2006). Communication with parents can focus on the child's positively developing skills and strengths. Child safety and communicable diseases are often topics of concern. Play groups allow parents to give each other support during these years.

School age (6–10 years)

These years are ones of phenomenal growth and development in many areas. Piaget described them as a period of 'concrete operations', meaning that logical thinking develops and the child can understand cause and effect. In the psychosocial realm, children are stimulated to become industrious and creative. Their vocabulary increases to 40,000 words, with reading supporting their verbal development (Berk 2006).

It is during the school years that many lifelong attitudes and values are shaped. For example, eating habits are formed and attitudes towards task accomplishment practised (Bastable 2006). A child who is not taught to use sunscreen and wear a hat outdoors may never value the health benefits of doing so. School-age children with chronic illnesses can be active in their own care because they understand the cause and effect related to taking medications or doing care activities like using inhalers. They can be included in patient teaching very effectively, as long as concrete methods are used such as pictures and demonstrations (Berk 2006). Parents can be helped to work with their child to understand an illness or injury and encourage the child to actively participate in care. Overprotection or condescending attitudes by adults can lead to feelings of inferiority and insecurity in the child.

The young person (10+ years)

Youth, teenage-hood and adolescence all evoke a time of major transition between childhood and adulthood. Physically, puberty brings about sometimes overwhelming hormonal transitions leading to alterations in how the young person functions socially and accepts themselves physically. Emotionally, there is the need for young people to separate themselves from parents and build their own identities (Bastable 2006).

A therapeutic relationship with a young person experiencing illness, injury or role confusion can be extremely valuable to future physical and emotional health. In a therapeutic relationship, a nurse can assist young people to explore their feelings, conflicts and personal dilemmas, as well as resources. Likewise, the parents of young people are vulnerable to feelings of conflict and separation anxiety and will find talking through these feelings very helpful (Groom et al. 2005). See Chapter 9 for further discussion of transition in the young person.

As with all developmental stages, there is no specific age at which the tasks of adolescence are completed. As young people begin employment and financial self-reliance, they also take more adult responsibilities upon themselves and yet may seem quite childlike in other respects. They may have difficulty with certain kinds of decisions or still engage in risky behaviours. If some of the psychosocial tasks of earlier stages have not been completed positively due to physical or emotional limitations or an unsupportive social environment, young people are especially vulnerable to disturbed behaviours (Groom et al. 2005). While physical maturity is fairly predictable on a chronological basis, emotional maturity is not. Young adults face many challenges in resolving what Erikson called intimacy versus isolation.

A therapeutic relationship with the young adult may engage not only with issues surrounding an illness, but also with issues such as career establishment, personal identity within an intimate relationship, and emotionally supportive alliances with family and friends. Continuing critical reflection as part of practice development will help nurses gain the self-awareness necessary to select those situations in which they can be helpful to patients and their families.

As suggested earlier, there can be an ethical dilemma presented to nurses who have intense relationships with more than one person in a family. Consider the example in Box 5.1.

Relationship development skills

Establishing a relationship with another person involves both the personal characteristics and skills of the nurse. In this section, both of these elements will be explored, as they contribute to the development of a therapeutic relationship. Mastery of communication skills is essential in making a thorough assessment of a person's needs and strengths and determining how the therapeutic relationship is to be focused.

Use of self to engage and encourage trust

In the earlier description of the characteristics of a therapeutic relationship, the 'use of self' was identified as especially important. This is a concept intrinsically linked

Box 5.1 Critical questions and reflections: therapeutic relationships with a teenager and her mother

Carla, aged 15 years, had been admitted to hospital with serious, but not life-threatening, injuries caused in a traffic accident in which a friend had been killed. One of the nurses, Julie, had formed a good therapeutic and helping relationship with her. They had some intense discussions about how Carla's injuries might affect her future life, her grief over her friend's death and how she was preparing for her dream of becoming a social worker. Julie had also established a good rapport with Carla's mother. They had explored Carla's ongoing needs and care as a result of her injuries and various issues of concern in raising a teenager.

Then one day Carla revealed that she and some friends had been experimenting with drugs just before the accident.

As Julie critically examines her feelings about this situation, she considers the following questions:

1. What is my professional responsibility related to information about drug use?
2. What are my ethical responsibilities related to confidentiality?
3. Should Carla be encouraged to tell her doctor and/or her mother about the drug use?
4. In what ways is Carla's care affected by my relationship with her mother?
5. In what ways is my relationship with Carla's mother affected by this information?
6. What would be your feeling if faced with this kind of dilemma? What resources are available to you in helping resolve it?

with caring—a central, if problematical, concept in nursing. Nurses often enter the profession because they intuitively know that 'caring' can make a difference in people's lives. But one might ask, what is caring and what personal characteristics does the nurse bring to caring relationships?

One way of looking at caring is to divide the activities of caring into three groups: use of the hands, use of the heart and use of the brain (Kapborg & Bertero 2003). Use of the hands is activity focused and means being physically present or caring 'for'. Use of the heart means being mentally and emotionally present or caring 'about'. Use of the brain means maintaining a professional perspective on the nurse–patient relationship and being aware of how the person of the nurse is affecting that relationship—in other words, caring 'with' (Shepherd 2001).

A therapeutic relationship seeks to achieve a trusting and enabling alliance and requires nurses to act from the heart and with intelligence and skill. Carl Rogers (1957) identified the helper's qualities of empathy, acceptance and genuineness as necessary for a therapeutic relationship. It is these latter terms that have become common in nursing, counselling and psychological literature. Whatever personal qualities are called, when they are perceived by another person, they are interpreted as concern and willingness to help. A nurse presents themselves to another person as trustworthy and willing to focus on the person's concerns and difficulties in an effort to resolve them. Although the phrase 'use of self' sounds rather contrived, engaging a person in a therapeutic relationship is a conscious and deliberate process. Through developed self-awareness, nurses allow themselves and their personal qualities to be known to a patient or family member. Using the 'core qualities' discussed by Rogers, here are some examples of how this works in practice.

Empathy

Empathy is the attempt to understand the needs and feelings of a person. It requires concentration to not just listen to words, but to hear what a person is saying. It also requires discipline to not interject one's own feelings or to respond with stories about situations in which the nurse felt the same way. For example, the father of a child in one's care remarks: 'I just feel so helpless!' It takes concentration to realise that this is a feeling that can be explored and perhaps turned into a plan, which helps the father feel more involved with his child. It takes discipline not to brush this comment away with false assurance such as, 'I know what you mean'.

In Harper Lee's (1960) novel, *To kill a mockingbird,* the main character is told how to get along with people. He is instructed to 'walk in their shoes'. Empathy means giving full attention to how it feels to be in someone else's shoes, not to join in the feelings (sympathy), but to try to understand at a deeply personal level.

Acceptance

Acceptance, sometimes termed respect, is non-judgmental. There is no power struggle when there is acceptance; the other person is recognised and appreciated as an equal. It is what Rogers meant by 'unconditional positive regard'. Age is not a barrier to acceptance and can be extended to children as well as adults of any age. Acceptance is demonstrating patience and concern for the person's experience. It is culturally sensitive, recognising that another person's experience might be quite different from one's own, but be just as valid (Stein-Parbury 2005). For example, acceptance is playing with or talking with a child until the child reaches out to be touched, rather than demanding a cuddle, which may well be rejected.

A nurse shows respect for a child's right to determine a comfortable level of physical contact. Acceptance is waiting for teenagers to sort through complex feelings, perhaps expressing half-formed descriptions before being ready to move towards self-awareness. Acceptance is allowing, even encouraging, the expression of strong emotions, even though that expression might make the nurse feel uncomfortable. Acceptance is kind, respectful, concerned and patient.

Genuineness

Being genuine is to be honest with oneself and others. It is to avoid verbal games or pretending to understand when one does not. This quality has also been termed authenticity or congruence (Stein-Parbury 2005). Genuineness means that the nurse's words, actions and intent are congruent, or in harmony, with one another. For example, genuineness is letting a person know that one is concerned about an issue, but that the pressure of work will not allow full attention to be given to it right now. Genuineness is letting a parent know that the nurse knows very little about a culture or religion, but is willing to listen and learn, and then taking steps to do so non-judgmentally.

When children or their families perceive empathy, acceptance and genuineness in a nurse's communication, they step towards trust in the carer and the care. In this way, a therapeutic relationship is in action.

Communication skills that build helping and therapeutic relationships

In addition to allowing oneself and one's personal qualities to be known to another person, the 'use of self' has to do with employing known communication methods that advance and sustain a therapeutic relationship. The nurse strives to develop inherent personal qualities through self-awareness. At the same time, the nurse strives to communicate well by learning and practising certain skills. In the following paragraphs, basic communication skills are outlined, including a variety of non-verbal means of communication and the effective use of questions and prompts.

Non-verbal skills

Non-verbal messages are critically important in establishing and maintaining a trust relationship. It is common experience that when a person's non-verbal behaviour does not agree with a spoken message, one accepts the non-verbal as honest (Stein-Parbury 2005). A nurse could say: 'I'm interested in your concerns'. If, at the same time, the nurse looks at the clock and seems to be restless, the message that the nurse has something more pressing to do than listen will be heard as true. Congruence between verbal and non-verbal behaviour demonstrates the nurse's genuineness and thereby encourages trust.

Focused attention in concentrated listening does not anticipate or interpret the meaning of what the person is saying, but simply pays attention to the here and now. It gives the nurse the opportunity not only to hear how people express themselves and their present concerns, but also allows observation of their level of congruence between non-verbal and verbal behaviour including tone of voice. The non-verbal aspect of communication is a window into the feelings that accompany the subject. For example, one can imagine the father who said he felt helpless saying these words in a slow, sad way, indicating his distress, or perhaps saying the words quickly with the pressure of anger, indicating his frustration.

Other aspects of non-verbal communication need to be considered in order to maintain and build effective communication with children and their families. Where children are involved, each of the following is a little different from interacting with adults and will need to be adapted to the child's age:

» *Posture*. It is important to maintain a relaxed open posture and be at the same height as the other person. This may involve sitting or crouching down.

» *Social distance*. Consider how far away to be to interact. Young babies, for example, have a short visual distance. Parents must be comfortable with the nurse's distance with them—about arm's length is appropriate, although this is culturally specific.

» *Touch*. Stranger intimacy is a concept that was developed in a seminal work by Jocalyn Lawler (1991) to describe the way in which nurses transgress usual conventions of both distance and touch in order to provide care. Consider appropriate and purposeful touch with different age children and in the context of caring for families.

» *Eye contact*. This is a culturally specific communication dynamic where the goal is to maintain respect and not be intrusive (Munoz & Luckman 2005).

» *Minimal encouragers*. These are responses that reflect what is being said without interrupting the flow of communication. They include repetition of significant words, gestures such as nods of the head, reflection of the feeling tone in the facial expressions of the listener, and sounds such as 'um-hmmm' (Ivey & Ivey 2003).

Using questions and prompts effectively

Nurses who have taken part in a basic communication skills course will know the difference between open and closed questions. Here is a brief summary:

» *Open questions* invite the person to explore the subject—for example, 'What is it you are most concerned about right now?' They suggest an openness to listening and for the other person to relate their story or concerns.

» *Prompts* are similar to open questions in that they invite exploration, but they may not be questions—for example, 'Tell me about . . .' (Stein-Parbury 2005).

» *Closed questions* seek specific information—for example, 'How long has Jeffrey been taking this medication?' Closed questions are effective for obtaining information quickly, as long as the right question is asked. They typically require only a short answer or a 'yes' or 'no' decision. They are, of course, useful for young children in that they can be used to discuss concrete activities. For example, an open question such as 'how are you feeling' may make sense to an adult as an invitation to describe symptoms, but to a young child it has little meaning. More effective may be a series of closed questions and prompts—for example, 'Does your leg hurt?' 'Point to the place it hurts.' 'Does it feel hot?'

To further develop your understanding of age-appropriate communication, consider the critical questions and reflections in Box 5.2.

Box 5.2 Critical questions and reflections: developing age-appropriate questions and prompts

Look back over the developmental challenges and phases of the various age groups of the child and young person. Develop a set of questions and prompts for each major age grouping designed to elicit initial information about presenting painful symptoms. Consider the input not only from the child, but also from family members.

Facilitating growth and change in therapeutic relationships

The goals of a therapeutic relationship are to facilitate the insight, growth and change that enable a person to build and use strengths and skills. This is the real 'work' of such a relationship. While every relationship is different in some respects, there are some key strategies nurses use in working with people to bring about that growth and change. Beginning with an assessment of strengths and resources, nurses may give support for change, inform and educate where additional knowledge or skill development is needed, and assist in bringing families and outside resources together. Each of these strategies is discussed in turn.

Assessing strengths and needs

In Chapter 1, comprehensive principles for family assessment and an approach to valuing and assessing family strengths are set out. The reader is referred to this chapter for more comprehensive information about family assessment. Other chapters throughout this text also provide insight into the way strengths-based approaches can be applied in nursing in specific child, youth and family settings.

Whatever the type of relationship, and the setting, nurses need to position themselves as a partner, instead of being seen as an expert who will attempt to 'fix' a problem situation. Assessment begins very early in a nurse–child or nurse–family relationship. A strengths-based approach to assessment is facilitative rather than directive, and anticipates positive outcomes through the mobilisation of resources and learning. In Box 5.3, an example of assessment based on a strengths approach is presented. It provides a simple example of strengths and resources and how these can be identified and utilised to support a family to meet their clinical and broader concerns by building on a family's experiences and helping them to reframe their expectations.

Box 5.3 Practice highlight: assessing strengths and resources in the complex care of an infant

Vania had cared for the infant Jamie for 2 days now following intestinal surgery. She had begun a good relationship with his mother, Janice. Vania knew that Jamie was a first child and that his care at home would be complex, involving regular tube feedings. In an effort to identify Janice's strengths and resources:

> *Vania:* 'Jamie was home for some time before he came in for this surgery. Can you tell me a bit about what that was like?'

> *Janice:* 'It wasn't easy, but my husband and I took turns getting up with him at night and the community nurse taught us some tricks to get him settled. We're pretty worried about how we're going to cope when he comes home this time.'

Vania noted the strength of cooperation between husband and wife and the resource of the community nurse. She was now able to give Janice some positive feedback about her and her husband working together and about her ability to use the community nurse's suggestions. Vania pointed out that the major difference in Jamie's care would be the tube feedings.

> *Janice:* 'It's good to know that his care won't be so very different. I am worried about the tube feedings. I've watched a couple of times, but I'll need practice before I can do them with anything like confidence.'

> *Vania:* 'That's really good you've taken the initiative in learning about Jamie's care.'

Vania then gave Janice a schedule of feeding times and reassurance that the nursing staff would be happy to help her learn.

Supportive intervention

The metaphor of a scaffold is a useful one to set out the kind of support offered by nurses within the context of a therapeutic relationship. Placed around a structure under construction, it provides support for change and development. It is not part of the structure, but purely temporary and will be removed when the structure is strong and able to function as intended. Like the scaffold, the nurse uses their knowledge and skills as a scaffold supporting, contributing information and skills, but keeping the focus on the patient or family member, and their needs.

Supportive intervention has as its goals encouraging emotional healing, building strengths and skills, maintaining self-esteem and promoting problem solving (Feeley & Gottlieb 2000). Like the builder on a scaffold, a nurse has a perspective on discrepancies in the structure. Gently pointing these out helps a person keep sight of important objectives. The nurse coaches, gives appropriate information and points the way forward in problem solving.

During assessment, nurses gather information and insight into family resources in order to guide supportive interventions. While strengths are internal to a family unit, resources exist externally and may be of several kinds (Feeley & Gottlieb 2000). Categories of resources include:

» material and financial resources
» social resources, such as extended family members, friends and neighbours, and
» professional resources, such as community health and human services.

An effective relationship and communication between nurse and family enables a family to identify the resources they have and how these may be helpful to them. Through effective communication and coordination, the nurse can assist a family to mobilise resources working with a family, at their level of knowledge and motivation. Availability, acceptability and accessibility are all critical aspects in mobilising resources.

Educational intervention

Educational interventions within the context of a therapeutic relationship are deliberate and focused. Using the earlier metaphor of the construction worker on a scaffold, the nurse brings the necessary materials to the building site. The materials must arrive at the appropriate level—that is, effective teaching builds on what is already known. They must also be timely—that is, the person must be receptive. Readiness develops out of the perception that learning will stimulate and reinforce the building process. Health literacy is about not only having information but also motivation, and means to utilise it to make changes (Nutbeam 2000).

Educational interventions may inform, develop a skill or encourage the development of positive attitudes. The discussion can centre on how the new information fits in with what the learner already knows or has experienced and how it can be used in the future. Demonstrations, written materials and pictures are helpful in reinforcing new knowledge, but are seldom effective when presented without iteration in discussion and interaction between nurse and learner.

Teaching methods and materials need to be adjusted according to the age and life experiences of the person, and literacy taken into account (Nutbeam 2000).

Young children need short, simple explanations. They relate to pictures and play. In one case, conjoined 4-year-old twins were given a doll similar to them to play with. They then performed 'surgery', separating the doll into two as a way of helping them understand the surgery that was planned for them.

Young people often relate well to examples from their own age group. Talking with another young person who has experienced a similar situation is often helpful. A teen diagnosed with diabetes will learn how to manage the disease better from another teen than from a lecture by the nurse. A nurse may take part or, alternatively, review the discussion with the young person in order to understand their comprehension and response to information and their situation and needs.

Whatever the primary purpose, effective communication using a range of interpersonal strategies and other tools is critical for good practice that is enabling to the child and their family.

Conclusion

This chapter has focused on communication in helping and therapeutic relationships specifically. Nurses deliberately use themselves, their personal characteristics, professional knowledge and communication skills to establish and maintain relationships with children, young people and their families in which both clinical information and feelings of health situations can be explored. The goals of therapeutic relationships are to enable the process of growth and change and, in so doing, to enable families to better meet the challenges of caring for children and young people and to make healthy decisions. Every therapeutic relationship is an opportunity for a nurse to develop self-awareness and professional skills. Critical reflection and practice development continue throughout a nurse's career and contribute significantly to a nurse's own self-esteem and career satisfaction.

Key points

- A therapeutic relationship focuses on both the clinical information and feelings of a health situation.
- Trust is a valuable quality in therapeutic relationships.
- In the care of children and young people, the focus of therapeutic relationships is the family.
- Understanding psychosocial, cognitive and emotional phases and challenges through infancy, childhood and into youth is essential in order to apply age-appropriate communication strategies.
- An emphasis on the strengths and resources of families allows the nurse to help them develop positive attitudes towards their capabilities.
- The nurse is a partner in helping to build strengths and resources.
- Supportive and educational interventions are used in working with families and are mediated through effective communication.
- The personal and communication skills demanded by effective therapeutic relationships are areas for career-long critical reflection and practice development.

Useful resources

Berk L 2006 *Child development*, 7th edn. Pearson, New York.
Better Health: www.betterhealth.vic.gov.au.
Early Childhood Connect: a website for the Centre for Health Equity, Training, Research and Evaluation, University of New South Wales, at http://chetre.med.unsw.edu.au/earlychildhood/index.htm. It has links to resources and research activities useful to nurses working in Australia.
Elder R, Evans K, Nizette D 2005 *Psychiatric and mental health nursing*. Elsevier, Sydney.
Stein-Parbury J 2005 *Patient and person: interpersonal skills in nursing*, 3rd edn. Elsevier, Sydney.

References

Australian Institute of Health and Welfare (AIHW) 2005 *Australia's welfare 2005*. AIWH, Canberra. Available at www.aihw.gov.au/.
Bastable SB 2006 *Essentials of patient education*. Jones & Bartlett, Sudbury, Massachusetts.
Berk L 2006 *Child development*, 7th edn. Pearson, New York.
Brammer L, MacDonald G 2003 *The helping relationship: process and skills*, 8th edn. Allyn & Bacon, Boston, Massachusetts.
DeFrain J 1999 Strong families around the world. *Family Matters* Winter 53:8.
Erikson EH 1963 *Childhood and society*, 2nd edn. Norton, New York.
Feeley N, Gottlieb L 2000 Nursing approaches for working with family strengths and resources. *Journal of Family Nursing* 6(1):9–24.
Gardner A, Goodsel J, Duggan T et al. 2001 'Don't call me sweetie!' Patients differ from nurses in their perceptions of caring. *Collegian* 8(3):32–8.
Graber DR, Mitcham MD 2004 Compassionate clinicians: taking patient care beyond the ordinary. *Holistic Nursing Practice* 18:87–94.
Groom M, Henderson K, Masters J 2005 Disorders of childhood and adolescence. In R Elder, K Evans & D Nizette (eds), *Psychiatric and mental health nursing*. Elsevier, Sydney, pp. 192–204.
Ivey A, Ivey M 2003 *Intentional interviewing and counseling*, 5th edn. Brooks/Cole, Pacific Grove, California.
Jackson D, Borbasi S-A 2000 The caring conundrum: potential and perils in nursing. In J Daly, S Speedy & D Jackson (eds), *Contexts of nursing: an introduction*. McLennan & Petty, Sydney.
Kapborg I, Bertero C 2003 The phenomenon of caring from the novice student nurse's perspective: a qualitative content analysis. *International Nursing Review* 50(3):183–92.
Lawler J 1991 *Behind the screens. Nursing, somology and the problem of the body*. Churchill Livingstone, Melbourne.
Lee H 1960 *To kill a mockingbird*. Harper Collins, New York.
McDevitt TM, Ormrod JE 2002 *Child development and education*. Pearson, Upper Saddle River, New Jersey.
McEwan M, Wills EM 2002 *Theoretical basis for nursing*. Lippincott Williams & Wilkins, Philadelphia.

Munoz C, Luckman J 2005 *Transcultural communication in nursing*. Thompson/Delmar Learning, Clifton Park, New York.

Nutbeam D 2000 Health literacy as a public health goal: a challenge for contemporary health education and communication strategies into the 21st century. *Health Promotion International* 15(3):259–67.

Piaget J 1951 *Judgment and reasoning in the child*. Routledge & Kegan Paul, London.

Rogers CR 1957 The necessary and sufficient conditions of therapeutic personality change. *Journal of Consulting Psychology* 21:95–103.

Shepherd M 2001 The healing power of professional invisibility. *Nuritinga* 4, June 2001. Available at www.healthsci.utas.edu.au.

Smith L 2002 Caring for the family. *Clinical Update*. Available at www.anj.org.au/04_anj_publications/anj_2002/0207_clin_update.pdf.

Stein-Parbury J 2005 *Patient and person: interpersonal skills in nursing*, 3rd edn. Elsevier, Sydney.

Part B

Practice contexts in child, youth and family health

Chapter 6

Pregnancy and birth: health and wellbeing for the woman and family

Cheryl Benn[1]

Learning outcomes

Reading this chapter will help you to:

- » describe the maternity care systems in Australia and New Zealand
- » identify at least four evidence-based practices for maintaining optimal health of the woman and her baby during pregnancy
- » define the concept 'health literacy' and apply the concept to antenatal preparation of parents
- » define attachment and describe the ways that attachment can be promoted in the early postnatal period
- » describe the key factors that can influence breastfeeding in the early postnatal period, and
- » discuss the impact on parents of giving birth to a preterm or sick baby.

Introduction

The decision to have a child or the discovery of pregnancy can be an exciting time for most women. It may also be challenging, depending on personal and social circumstances. It initiates a complex set of changes and transitions, which impact on the individuals in a family in dramatic and sometimes unrecognised ways. A healthy pregnancy and good preparation for the important parenting transitions and family

1 We would like to acknowledge the contribution of Margaret Barnes to the final version of this chapter.

adjustments ahead are critical to ensure the best health and wellbeing of the woman, her child, her partner and other family. The challenges are biophysical, emotional and psychosocial, woven in complex webs in a woman's life.

In this chapter, women's health in pregnancy, maternity services, options for antenatal care and birth, as well as parenting preparation, are discussed. In addition, attention is given to preterm birth, an experience that creates unique and significant stressors and vulnerabilities for the health and wellbeing of childbearing women and their families.

Setting the scene: a clinical scenario

This scenario introduces us to a woman early in her third pregnancy. It shows some of the challenges pregnant women and their families encounter, and the numerous, and at times, unplanned, pathways they follow towards the birth of a child.

Kay, aged 37, and her partner Richard, aged 40, live in Auckland. They are expecting a baby. Kay has two children from a previous relationship—Scotty, aged 8, and Oliver, aged 6, both born at term, in hospital. Early in this pregnancy Kay and Richard chose a midwife as their lead maternity carer. They are hoping that they may be able to have a homebirth.

All progressed well until at 33 weeks Kay's waters broke and she went into spontaneous labour. She was admitted to the maternity unit. Her baby was born vaginally, weighing 1875 grams, and was transferred to the neonatal special care nursery.

The context of maternity care in Australia and New Zealand

Kay and Richard had health provider options available to support Kay's pregnancy and were in a position to make a choice. Service organisations in New Zealand and Australia are quite distinct.

In New Zealand, the maternity system requires a woman to choose a health professional to be her Lead Maternity Carer (LMC), and in some areas this person may be a midwife, a general practitioner or an obstetrician. Rural areas and some provincial towns do not have all these types of practitioners available to provide LMC, so the choice is limited for those women. However, currently over 80% of women choose a midwife as their LMC (Guilliland 2006).

The important principles underpinning maternity services in New Zealand include, first, a commitment to primary healthcare, provided in the home or hospital, and, second, continuity of care by a known/named caregiver through pregnancy, childbirth and the postnatal period to 4–6 weeks postpartum, supported by secondary and tertiary services (Ministry of Health New Zealand 2000, MidCentral Health District Health Board 2005). Further, maternity services are underpinned by the key principles of informed decision making and informed consent.

In Australia, private and public maternity health service options are available. Women may attend for antenatal care with their general practitioner or at a health service such as a local hospital or clinic. Many health services offer midwifery-led care, but this varies from service to service and state to state. Women may choose to contract a midwife working in private practice for their maternity care, but at a cost to themselves.

While options for midwifery-led care have expanded, equitable access to one-to-one maternity care is not available for all women, a situation that has led to a number of political actions. For example, Maternity Coalition has developed a *National maternity action plan* for the introduction of services in rural and regional Australia (www.maternitycoalition.org.au/), and, more recently, a review of birthing services in Queensland has highlighted the need for maternity care reform in Australia (Hirst 2005). There is research evidence that this one-to-one kind of service by a known health professional provides clear benefits for women during pregnancy and childbirth, an issue which is discussed further later in this chapter (Hodnett 2000, Hildingsson et al. 2002).

Hospital or home: an issue of safety?

For Kay and Richard, the place of birth for their baby was important. After two uncomplicated hospital births, Kay and Richard planned a birth at home with a midwife as LMC provider. However, the early labour required a change of plan.

Looking back to the early 1900s, most women in New Zealand and other parts of the world gave birth at home (Banks 2000, Tew 1990). The rise of public health initiatives and health surveillance led to, first, antenatal clinics and lying-in wards and, finally, the normalisation of hospital as the safe place to give birth. The notion of the hospital as a safe birthing place has been critiqued (Tew 1990). In the 1990s, a number of studies examined the relative safety of birth settings (Bateman et al. 1994, Berghs et al. 1995, Truffert et al. 1998, Waldenstrom & Nilsson 1997). A recent systematic review regarding home/homelike versus hospital or conventional institutional settings for birth concluded that homelike settings were associated with reduced medical interventions and increased maternal satisfaction. They did warn however that 'caregivers and clients should be vigilant for signs of complications' (Hodnett et al. 2005 p. 1).

The important points from the Hodnett et al. (2005) review indicate that women labour better and are more satisfied with the outcomes and the care received when in homelike settings. Homelike settings were described as relaxed, where there were no routine interventions, dress code or expectations. Women were able to move around freely and adopt any position they wished. Continuity of carer is also important in this setting, with no time constraints such as those imposed by institutions with strict protocols.

One of the advantages of homebirth settings over homelike settings is that the woman is in her own home and the professional is a guest, who decides when she needs to hand over or transfer care. The midwife also attends when the woman decides she wants her to do so. This kind of environment means there are fewer interventions and the woman is not constrained to 'perform' according to a specified timeline. Debate continues on this issue and looks set to do so for some time yet. To explore further the issue of continuity, see Box 6.1.

Box 6.1 Practice highlight: continuity of care

The terms 'continuity of care' and 'continuity of caregiver' have been differentiated by some practitioners as being equally acceptable or meaning the same thing. However, an examination of the extant literature reveals some subtle differences. Continuity of care would be the care provided by different caregivers, but with a good overview of the woman's history and pregnancy to date through the use of clinical records (Medical Records Institute 2006), while continuity of caregiver is defined as care provided by one person or a small group of caregivers through the maternity or illness experience (Haggerty et al. 2003).

Other terms used to describe this relationship were found by Haggerty et al. who were commissioned by the Canadian health services and policy research bodies to develop a common understanding of the concept of continuity. The additional terms include 'longitudinality', 'relational' or 'personal continuity' (p. 1219). Buetow (2004) borrowed the terms 'informational continuity' and 'relational or interpersonal continuity' from Haggerty et al. (2003), but challenged the fact that continuity of caregiver is focused on the *one* carer who is usually a health professional rather than on *all* those involved in care, such as family members, who will ask questions on behalf of, listen to information provided and provide ongoing supportive care in the absence of the health professional.

There is good evidence (Hodnett 2000, Hildingsson et al. 2002) that continuity of caregiver does make a positive difference to women's attendance of antenatal classes, their use of analgesia in labour and the resuscitation required by their newborns. However, Hodnett (2000) does indicate that it is not clear from the two major studies that were included in the systematic review undertaken whether the differences were due to continuity of caregiver or the fact that the caregiver was a midwife. Hildingsson et al. (2002) in their survey of Swedish women attending for antenatal care found that the 91% of women who responded ($N = 3061$) appreciated the system of continuity of midwife carer during pregnancy.

Critical question: barriers and restraints

1. As continuity of carer is considered to have positive impacts on the health and wellbeing of women and their families, what are the barriers and constraints to implementing such care in mainstream maternity services?

Health promotion during pregnancy

Promoting a woman's health in pregnancy influences perinatal outcomes and antenatal care has become a central focus of professional support for pregnant women and their families. However, antenatal care is a twentieth century phenomenon, which was first introduced by means of pro-maternity hospitals set up by Dr JW Ballantyne for women who were ill and tired in pregnancy, but primarily for doctors to learn more about the mother and fetus during pregnancy (Tew 1990).

The first outpatient clinic for pregnant women was established in 1911 in the United States, followed by similar clinics in Britain in 1915 and later in other parts of the world. Antenatal care from the 1960s onwards was seen as a means of reducing and preventing fetal death and handicap, rather than reducing maternal mortality.

The World Health Organization (2005) recommends that effective and appropriate antenatal care be offered to all women; however, it questions some of the practices and interventions included. Some interventions offered to women with a low-risk pregnancy are not effective, while many others have not been evaluated, such as the timing and type of antenatal visits that may be most effective (Enkin et al. 2000).

Antenatal care has been cited as ritualistic rather than rational (Enkin et al. 2000). One systematic review of literature concerning antenatal visiting patterns suggests that while a smaller number of visits may be more effective than the number traditionally suggested, women are less satisfied with less rather than more (Villar et al. 2001, Villar & Khan-Neelofur 2001). In Box 6.2, selected evidence-based practices are described.

Box 6.2 Practice highlight: maintaining optimal health and wellbeing during pregnancy—selected evidence-based practices

- Attend for antenatal care regularly. However, the schedule of appointments should be individualised and have a specific focus rather than just following a routine schedule (National Collaborating Centre for Women's and Children's Health 2003).
- Women-held antenatal records improves clinical safety, wellbeing and women's sense of control (Brown & Smith 2004, Elbourne et al. 1987, Homer et al. 1999).
- Women should be informed of the symptoms of advanced pre-eclampsia, such as any visual disturbances, epigastric pain, vomiting and increasing oedema, and the need to report them early to their care provider (National Collaborating Centre for Women's and Children's Health 2003).
- Screen for risk factors for pre-eclampsia at the first antenatal visit and schedule visits according to identified risks (National Collaborating Centre for Women's and Children's Health 2003).
- Women should be encouraged to report decreased movements to their healthcare provider. However, there is no evidence that routine monitoring of fetal movements prevents late fetal deaths (National Collaborating Centre for Women's and Children's Health 2003). A systematic review is currently being undertaken by Mangesi and Hofmeyr (2004 p. 2) 'to assess the outcome of pregnancy when fetal movement is done routinely, selectively, or not at all and using various methods'.
- Symphysis–fundal height should be measured and plotted at each antenatal appointment (National Collaborating Centre for Women's and Children's Health 2003). This is a recommended method of assessing fetal growth, as opposed to the formerly used method of routine weighing of pregnant women.

Preconception and pregnancy health

Ideally, women and their partners will consider their health and lifestyle prior to pregnancy. The aim of preconception health and care is to identify and if possible modify biomedical, behavioural and social risks to a woman's health and prospective pregnancy (Centers for Disease Control 2006). The focus of preconception care is to screen for risks, engage in health promotion and education, and intervene when risks are identified (Centers for Disease Control 2006).

The key areas of concern during the preconception period include:

» assessment of general health and wellbeing, including nutrition and exercise patterns

» management of existing disorders (e.g. diabetes)
» screening and vaccination, if necessary, against rubella
» folic acid supplementation to reduce the risk of neural tube defects
» smoking cessation counselling, to reduce the risk of low birth weight and other adverse perinatal outcomes
» recommending abstinence from alcohol to prevent fetal alcohol syndrome and other alcohol-related birth defects
» review of medication use, and
» sexually transmitted disorders screening to reduce risks to mother and fetus (Centers for Disease Control 2006).

Preconception care helps ensure that the woman entering pregnancy is in good health with as few risk factors as possible, which will optimise maternal and perinatal outcomes (Moos 2003). However, the majority of women receive fragmented care throughout the childbearing period and often will only attend for care when there are signs of a pregnancy. Moos (2003) suggests a continuum model of integrated care for women, where health providers build on what is learned about a woman's health and integrate health promotion opportunistically, prior to pregnancy. In this model, all women who are of reproductive age benefit from care and information that will influence their health at the time of a pregnancy. Cullum (2003) suggests that preconception refers to that time when a woman is fertile, but not pregnant, widening the potential for healthcare and health promotion among women prior to pregnancy.

Why health and wellbeing in, before and during pregnancy is important

At the heart of preconception and pregnancy care is the proposition that optimising the health of mother and fetus will influence not only perinatal outcomes, but also the infant's health in adult life. Important to this understanding is the influence of social as well as physical health during the reproductive years. The practice highlight in Box 6.3 describes two selected health issues for women to consider before and during pregnancy.

The way in which social and physical health are interrelated is highlighted through an understanding of the fetal origins hypothesis. Proposed by Barker in 1998, this hypothesis suggests that infants born following fetal growth retardation and, therefore, of low birth weight, are at increased risk for developing cardiovascular and diabetic disease later in life (Barker 2003). In addition to biophysical factors, there are many social determinants of low birth weight, and thus the importance of health promoting activities focused on healthy pregnancy are made clear.

Spencer (2000 p. 194) suggests:

> '. . . the birth weight of an infant reflects quality of the fetal environment and the length of gestation, which are influenced by intergenerational, genetic, constitutional, dietary and lifestyle factors. It is a pivotal point in the life-course continuum reflecting maternal health and predicting future health in childhood and adulthood.'

Box 6.3 Practice highlight: preconception and pregnancy care

Substance use in pregnancy

The use of substances such as alcohol, nicotine via cigarette smoking or nicotine patch or gum use, or other toxins via marijuana smoking or the use of other illegal or prescribed drugs, is considered potentially harmful to the developing baby. The fetus is also particularly vulnerable during the first 3–8 weeks of pregnancy, and may be at risk of being born preterm or of low birth weight. These babies may also suffer from drug withdrawal and conditions known as fetal alcohol syndrome (FAS) or to a lesser extent a range of effects grouped under the term fetal alcohol spectrum disorder (FASD) and/or fetal tobacco syndrome, which will affect their long-term cognitive abilities and behaviours. Substance use and abuse often leads to poor nutrition in pregnancy (Parackal 2003). In the case of alcohol abuse, this may be because of the energy derived from the alcohol or because of economic or lifestyle constraints related to a high alcohol intake.

Folate in pregnancy and breastfeeding

Folate is a generic term applied to dietary sources of related compounds involved in the metabolism of nucleic and amino acids. They are expressed as Dietary Folate Equivalents (DFE), which includes folate from food and folic acid which is a synthetic form of folate (Ministry of Health New Zealand 2006). Folates are especially important during pregnancy and breastfeeding when nucleotide synthesis and cell division are occurring, and have been associated with a decrease in the incidence of neural tube defects, the most common congenital abnormality (Boddie et al. 2000).

Critical questions: smoking cessation

1. Review the literature related to smoking cessation in pregnancy.
2. Which strategies have been successful and which have not been so successful?

Such interconnected factors influence the fetal and early childhood environment and may provide protection or place the child at risk.

Pregnancy is a time when opportunities for health promotion present themselves, not only for the woman and family in this pregnancy and birth, but also for long-term health. One strategy used to frame this health promotion has been antenatal education.

Antenatal education

Nolan (1997) suggests that antenatal education is not new—women previously and still do learn about pregnancy and birth from their female relatives and friends. Nolan (1997) suggests that antenatal education is an artificial construct aiming to replace the knowledge and insights traditionally transmitted among women. This replacement has, however, not been entirely successful.

Antenatal classes have traditionally focused on preparing the couple or woman for labour and birth, but new parents are increasingly voicing their concerns about the lack of preparation for actual parenting—the most important and long-term role that results from a pregnancy (Ho & Holroyd 2002). While antenatal education is constantly evaluated and changing, much of the class time is spent covering topics such as pain management and obstetric interventions.

In addition, the needs of young teenage mothers and sometimes their partners may not be addressed through mainstream antenatal classes, as they are often aimed at older women in partnered relationships. The classes, and the teachers, need to be innovative and flexible so as to be able to address the needs of individuals and couples as they arise over the course of the classes. However, despite many decades of development in the field of antenatal education, the effects of general antenatal education for childbirth and/or parenthood remain unknown (Gagnon 2000, World Health Organization 2005).

As a result of time limitations and a focus on a set curriculum aimed at preparing women and their partners for labour and birth, the main function of antenatal classes seems to be information transfer rather than to improve health literacy. Health literacy is a concept that has been in the literature for over 30 years (Nutbeam 2000, Renkert & Nutbeam 2001), but to a large extent has been very narrowly defined as being focused on 'the ability to apply literacy skills to health related materials such as prescriptions, appointment cards' (Nutbeam 2000 p. 263). The World Health Organization defines health literacy much more broadly, indicating that 'by improving people's access to health information and their capacity to use it effectively, health literacy is critical to empowerment' (Nutbeam 1998 p. 357).

A shift in focus from information provision to improving health literacy should therefore be the goal of all antenatal education, and, as many women and partners do not attend formal classes, an emphasis on education and discussion during antenatal care visits may be more beneficial. Indeed, the most important benefit of formal classes may be the opportunity to develop a social network (Fabian et al. 2005) with other women and partners in the same life stage. As it is often midwives and nurses who are involved in the preparation and presentation of antenatal education, this is a key area for consideration.

Applying these principles to the scenario, it is clear that Kay and Richard have made choices about this pregnancy based on their previous experiences and information they have accessed. Their planning for a birth at home and choice of a midwife LMC were based on well-considered and informed decisions. They recognised the benefits of having one professional provide continuity of care. While their plans needed to change, Kay and Richard were motivated, well informed and felt included in the decision-making process, even though they were disappointed about such an unexpected outcome.

The transition following birth

Birth is a significant life event that initiates a sequence of changes and transitions, perhaps like no other during the life course. This transition is a major change for the woman, her partner and family. During this time, a woman as primary carer, but also her partner and other family members, have to get to know the baby, how the baby behaves, what these behaviours might mean, as well as providing basic care that provides for the baby's needs, warmth, comfort and contact, and food. Basic skills in caring for a baby such as hygiene, changing nappies, feeding, and preventing distress and crying, are learned in the early weeks after birth. Learning to determine whether a baby is healthy or sick is another challenge for new parents who may be afraid of overreacting and seeking care too early or more so of underreacting and seeking care only when it is too late.

Women and their partners have to adjust to changes in their own relationships and everyday habits and rituals, such as sleep patterns. Changes to relationships occur during this important transition time. Fatigue after the birth and in the early days and weeks of parenting are often cited by women as reasons for not needing or wanting to be close to their partner. It is all these tasks that not only need to be learned, but also need time for the psychological adaptation or transition to occur (Bridges 2004). To examine the role of fathers and partners in the transition following birth, consider the critical questions and reflections in Box 6.4.

Box 6.4 Critical questions and reflections: transition to fatherhood

Fatherhood and fathering only began to attract significant scholarly attention in the 1990s. This trend reflects changing social patterns where both domestic and public organisation of families have been changing. In order to learn more about men's experiences as they make the transition to fatherhood, conduct a search using nursing and social science databases to find at least five papers that focus on this topic. Read these and develop a summary of fatherhood transition challenges for:

1. identity
2. parenting competence, and
3. everyday lifestyle.

The importance of attachment

Attachment is the development of the strong relationship between a mother or a caregiver and a baby, which leads to emotional security in the child. Bowlby (1969) observed infant–caregiver relationships and interactions, and theorised that the initial relationship is based on a set of innate signals that call the caregiver to the infant's side and that during the first year of life a true affectionate bond develops.

The importance of attachment was first signalled through the work of Bowlby (1969) and Ainsworth (1962), as well as more current thinking as highlighted in the World Health Organization document on the importance of caregiver–child interactions (2004). Bowlby, in his early work, emphasised the importance and the primacy of interpersonal relationships for young children and suggested that the formation of such relationships was as important to child survival as food, stimulation and physical care (World Health Organization 2004). Further, Erikson (n.d. p. 51) suggests that 'although not an inoculation against later problems, secure attachment in infancy lays the foundation for healthy development'.

Recent evidence suggests that it is not only social and psychological wellbeing that is influenced by secure attachment, but that children's neurological development occurs in response to social and interpersonal processes (Nelson & Bloom 1997,

Schore 2001). The infant's brain has been described as being experience-dependent and experience-expectant in that new synaptic connections occur in response to experiences. Therefore, an infant's development is dependent upon sensory and motor stimulation (experiences) from caregivers, a kind of stimulation that occurs during affective interactions with responsive caregivers (World Health Organization 2004).

Attachment and skin-to-skin contact

While the interaction between the infant and caregiver needs to be consistent and long term, the experience around birth and the early postnatal period provides an opportunity to establish this relationship early. A mother's responsiveness to the signals from her baby is strongly influenced by the immediate postbirth period and the opportunities she is afforded to hold and get to know her baby undisturbed. It is therefore important to establish a birthing environment that encourages immediate and close contact.

One way in which attachment in the immediate postbirth period can be encouraged is via skin-to-skin contact, whether the baby is born full or preterm. Significant and positive effects of early contact on breastfeeding at 1–3 months postbirth, and on breastfeeding duration, and improved maternal attachment behaviours, have been found to be associated with skin-to-skin contact (Anderson et al. 2003).

For Kay, Richard and their infant, this undisturbed contact following birth is only possible for a short period. However, every effort is made to reduce times of separation and to help Kay initiate breastfeeding. In the context of premature birth, Kangaroo Mother Care (KMC) has become a widely adopted approach to increasing the close contact of infant with mother. KMC was first proposed in Colombia in 1978 in response to hospital overcrowding and resource scarcity, and mimics marsupial caregiving. KMC was found to have physiological benefits for the baby as well as for the parent–child relationship. It has been shown that KMC mothers feel more competence in their caregiving than mothers of infants nursed solely in incubators, particularly over longer periods of hospitalised care (Tessier et al. 1998).

Parents require significant support for KMC, initiating breastfeeding or expressing breastmilk if their infant is not able to feed, and other activities if their parenting transitions are to be facilitated in this care environment.

Parenting preterm newborns

Parenting in neonatal nurseries is stressful, and hinders parent–infant attachment and the development of parenting competence. The emotions that mothers and fathers of preterm infants experience may include:

» *Emotional trauma and guilt*. They may ask what they did to cause the premature birth. They feel guilt because they want to be with their baby in the neonatal nursery, but their older children also need them.

» *Shock*. The outcome may have been unexpected and very sudden.

» *Grief*. Grief may be experienced because of unmet expectations (Booth & Bartle 2005).

Adapting to risk, protecting fragility, preserving the family, compensating for the past and cautiously affirming the future are all themes that have been identified as impacting on parenting perceptions of this time (Schwarz 2005). Supporting parents in this technologically intense environment helps to reduce their stress (Whitfield 2003). Family-centred supportive care is an important practice for nurses (Miles et al. 1996, Holditch-Davis & Miles 2000, Cox & Bialoskurski 2001, Fenwick et al. 2001, Cescutti-Butler & Galvin 2003), and yet is challenging in the intense and medically focused neonatal nursery care environment. Nurses need to share information with parents and engage them as partners in caregiving and decision making (Griffin 2006). Anticipatory guidance and education is thought to enable the parents to cope with their 'at risk' children (Schwarz 2005). The issues facing parents of preterm infants are explored further in Chapter 12, with Tihema and her family.

Supporting breastfeeding

Initiating breastfeeding in the postnatal period is of critical importance to attachment and to the health and wellbeing of an infant in both the short and longer term. Supporting breastfeeding is a key health promotion activity as the benefits of breastfeeding for infant, mother, family and community are well-recognised.

Breastfeeding is recognised as the optimal method of infant feeding and confers a number of health benefits, including reduced incidence of gastrointestinal illness (Kramer & Kakuma 2003), respiratory illness, asthma and allergies (Oddy et al. 1999, Gdalevich et al. 2001).

Breastfeeding may protect against the development of obesity (von Kries et al. 1999) and development of illness in later life (e.g. type 2 diabetes and cardiovascular disease) (Pettitt et al. 1997, Bergstrom et al. 1995). Current breastfeeding initiation rates in Australia and New Zealand are relatively high. Figures suggest that rates stabilised in the 1990s, and, in 2001, were about 83% (Australian Bureau of Statistics 2003, Ministry of Health New Zealand 2002).

However, there are a number of factors that influence a woman's decision to breastfeed and her ability to continue breastfeeding during the infant's first year. Factors such as socioeconomic status (Donath & Amir 2000), lower maternal education and father's occupational status, as well as having a caesarean section and infant admission to special care nursery, are cited as having a negative impact on breastfeeding (Scott et al. 2001). Breastfeeding rates at 3 and 6 months are significantly lower than the initiation rate, and programs to assist women to continue breastfeeding are constantly evaluated. These issues are explored further in Chapter 7. While many factors influence the initiation and maintenance of breastfeeding, one example is provided in the research highlight in Box 6.5.

Assisting women to understand and manage breastfeeding and lactation during pregnancy and in the postnatal period is important to subsequent breastfeeding success. Practices that facilitate and support breastfeeding are outlined in the 'Ten steps to successful breastfeeding' (UNICEF/World Health Organization 2006), which are listed in Box 6.6. Implementation of these practices as routine ensures that maternity service environments promote, support and protect breastfeeding, and consider breastfeeding as the 'norm'.

Box 6.5 Research highlight: epidurals and breastfeeding

There is a growing body of evidence (Murray et al. 1981, Abboud et al. 1982, Jordan et al. 2005, Riordan 1999, Beilin et al. 2005, Torvaldsen et al. 2006) that epidurals in labour have an impact on a baby's ability to exhibit early neurobehaviours, such as rooting, sucking and state organisation, that will facilitate successful breastfeeding. While Torvaldsen et al. (2006) comment that no causal link can be established between an epidural with fentanyl as an opioid during labour and successful breastfeeding, they do emphasise the need for increased breastfeeding assistance and support for women who have had such an epidural during labour.

However, Beilin et al. (2005) in a randomised, double blind study also found that women with previous experience of breastfeeding, who had an epidural in labour with high does of fentanyl as compared with low doses or no fentanyl, were more likely to have babies with low neurobehaviour scores and to have stopped breastfeeding at 6 weeks postpartum.

Practice points

1. Give women full information about types of analgesia and their effects in labour and on breastfeeding.
2. Provide extra support and assistance with breastfeeding to women who have had epidurals in labour.
3. Use other non-pharmacological forms of pain relief before resorting to any pharmacological forms.

Box 6.6 Practice highlight: practices that protect, support and promote breastfeeding

The 10 steps to successful breastfeeding (UNICEF/World Health Organization 2006) are:

1. Have a written breastfeeding policy that is routinely communicated to all healthcare staff.
2. Train all healthcare staff in skills necessary to implement this policy.
3. Inform all pregnant women about the benefits and management of breastfeeding.
4. Help mothers initiate breastfeeding within a half-hour of birth.
5. Show mothers how to breastfeed and how to maintain lactation even if they should be separated from their infants.
6. Give newborn infants no food or drink other than breastmilk, unless medically indicated.
7. Practice rooming-in. Allow mothers and infants to remain together—24 hours a day.
8. Encourage breastfeeding on demand.
9. Give no artificial teats or pacifiers (also called dummies or soothers) to breastfeeding infants.
10. Foster the establishment of breastfeeding support groups and refer mothers to them on discharge from the hospital or clinic.

Reader activity

Consider the 10 steps and identify the ways in which these practices could be integrated for Kay and her baby.

Conclusion

In this chapter, the focus was on the health services available to support a pregnant woman through her pregnancy and into the immediate postnatal period. The importance of health promotion and the role of the midwife and nurse were explored with a focus on some of the evidence for and against particular practices. Health professionals have a vital role to play in providing parents with information and skills that will enable them to make informed decisions about pregnancy care, birth and postnatal care. Shifting the emphasis in antenatal care and education to an approach that improves health literacy is suggested as a strategy for improving decision making for this group.

Practice tips

- Promote good nutrition and healthy lifestyle choices.
- Encourage continuity of caregiver to ensure improved outcomes for mothers and babies.
- Include all members of the family in the consultations and visits to promote continuity of care.
- Individualise the care provided during pregnancy, labour, birth and postpartum.
- Provide information to assist parents to make informed choices and decisions about their healthcare needs and those of their infants.
- Health literacy will empower the developing family to seek and find information to meet their health needs.
- Keep mother and baby together, preferably skin-to-skin after birth.
- Delay any routine interventions and practices as far as possible.
- Protect, support and promote breastfeeding.
- Fully involve the mother and father in the care of a preterm or sick newborn baby.

Useful resources

Australian Institute of Health and Welfare (AIHW) 2004 *Australia's mothers and babies 2004*. Available at www.aihw.gov.au/riskfactors/overweight.cfm.

Circle of Security: www.circleofsecurity.org/.

National Collaborating Centre for Women's and Children's Health 2003 *Antenatal care. Routine care for the healthy pregnant woman. Clinical guideline*. Available at www.rcog.org.uk/resources/Public/pdf/Antenatal_Care.pdf.

National maternity action plan: www.maternitycoalition.org.au/.

New Zealand Health Information Service (NZHIS) 2006 *Report on maternity: maternity and newborn information 2003*. Available at www.nzhis.govt.nz/stats/index.html.

World Health Organization (WHO) 2002 *Essential newborn care and breastfeeding. Training modules*. WHO, Geneva. Available at www.euro.who.int/document/e79227.pdf.

World Health Organization (WHO) 2005 *What is the effectiveness of antenatal care?* (Supplement). WHO, Geneva. Available at www.euro.who.int/Document/E87997.pdf.

References

Abboud TK, Klaas SS, Miller F et al. 1982 Maternal, fetal, and neonatal responses after epidural anesthesia with bupivacaine, 2-chloroprocaine, or lidocaine. *Anesthetic Analgesia* 61:638–44.

Ainsworth M 1962 The effects of maternal deprivation: a review of findings and controversy in the context of research strategy. In MSD Ainsworth, RG Andry & RG Harlow et al. (eds), *Deprivation of maternal care: a reassessment of its effects*. World Health Organization, Geneva.

Anderson GC, Moore E, Hepworth J, Bergman N 2003 *Early skin-to-skin contact for mothers and their healthy newborn infants (review)*. Cochrane Database of Systematic Reviews. Issue 2, Art. No. CD003519. DOI: 10.1002/14651858. CD003519.

Australian Bureau of Statistics (ABS) 2003. *Breastfeeding in Australia 2001*. Available at www.abs.gov.au/AUSSTATS/abs @.nsf/cat/4810.0.55.001.

Banks M 2000 *Homebirth bound: mending the broken weave*. Birthspirit Books, Hamilton, New Zealand.

Barker D 2003 The midwife, the coincidence, and the hypothesis. *British Medical Journal* 327:1428–30.

Bateman DA, O'Bryan L, Nicholas SW, Heagarty MC 1994 Outcome of unattended out-of-hospital births in Harlem. *Archives of Pediatric and Adolescent Medicine* 148:147–52.

Beilin Y, Bodian CA, Weiser J et al. 2005 Effect of labour epidural analgesia with and without fentanyl on infant breast-feeding: a prospective, randomized, double-blind study. *Anethesiology* 103(6):1211–17.

Berghs G, Spanjaards E, Driessen L et al. 1995 Neonatal neurological outcome after low-risk pregnancies. *European Journal of Obstetrics & Gynaecology and Reproductive Biology* 62(2):167–71.

Bergstrom E, Hernell O, Persson LA, Vessby B 1995 Serum lipid values in adolescents are related to family history, infant feeding and physical growth. *Atherosclerosis* 117(1):1–13.

Boddie AM, Dedlow ER, Nackashi JA et al. 2000 Folate absorption in women with a history of neural tube defect-affected pregnancy. *American Journal of Clinical Nutrition* 72(1):154–8.

Booth D, Bartle C 2005 NUMB Neonatal unity for mothers and babies. *CENZ Effect* 3:9–11.

Bowlby J 1969 *Attachment and loss. Vol. 1. Attachment*. Basic Books, New York.

Bridges W 2004 *Transitions: making sense of life's changes*. De Capo Press, Cambridge, Mass.

Brown HC, Smith HJ 2004 *Giving women their own case notes to carry during pregnancy*. Cochrane Database of Systematic Reviews. Issue 2, Art. No. CD002856.

Buetow SA 2004 Towards a new understanding of provider continuity. *Annals of Family Medicine* 2(5):509–11.

Centers for Disease Control (CDC) 2006 *Preconception health and care*. Department of Health and Human Services, Atlanta.

Cescutti-Butler L, Galvin K 2003 Parents' perceptions of staff competency in a neonatal intensive care unit. *Journal of Clinical Nursing* 12:752–61.

Cox C, Bialoskurski M 2001 Neonatal intensive care: communication and attachment. *British Journal of Nursing* 10:668–76.

Cullum A 2003 Changing provider practices to enhance preconceptional wellness. *Journal of Obstetric, Gynecologic and Neonatal Nursing* 32(4):543–9.

Donath S, Amir LH 2000 Rates of breastfeeding in Australia by state and socio-economic status: evidence from the 1995 National Health Survey. *Journal of Paediatrics and Child Health* 36:164–8.

Elbourne D, Richardson M, Chalmers I et al. 1987 The Newbury maternity care study: a randomized controlled trial to assess a policy of women holding their own obstetric records. *British Journal of Obstetrics and Gynaecology* 94:612–19.

Enkin M, Keirse MJNC, Neilson J et al. 2000 *A guide to effective care in pregnancy and childbirth*, 3rd edn. Oxford University Press, Oxford.

Erikson MF n.d. Building resiliency and reducing risk. Wisconsin Family Impact Seminars. Available at http://familyimpactseminars.org/fis10erickson.htm. Accessed 22 February 2007.

Fabian H, Rådestad I, Waldenström U 2005 Childbirth and parenthood education classes in Sweden. Women's opinion and possible outcomes. *Acta Obstetricia et Gynecologica Scandinavica* 84:436–43.

Fenwick J, Barclay L, Schmied V 2001 'Chatting': an important clinical tool in facilitating mothering in neonatal nurseries. *Journal of Advanced Nursing* 33:583–93.

Gagnon AJ 2000 *Individual or group antenatal education for childbirth/parenthood.* Cochrane Database of Systematic Reviews. Issue 4, Art. No. CD002869.

Gdalevich M, Mimouni D, Mimouni M 2001 Breastfeeding and the risk of bronchial asthma in childhood: a systematic review with a meta-analysis of prospective studies. *Journal of Pediatrics* 139(2):261–6.

Griffin T 2006 Family-centred care in the NICU. *Journal of Perinatal and Neonatal Nursing* 20(1):98–102.

Guilliland K 2006 The media can make up the story but prejudice fuels it. *Midwifery News* 40:7.

Haggerty JL, Reid RJ, Freeman GK et al. 2003 Continuity of Care: a multidisciplinary review. *British Medical Journal* 327:1219–21.

Hildingsson I, Waldenström U, Rådestad I 2002 Women's expectations on antenatal care as assessed in early pregnancy: number of visits, continuity of caregiver and general content. *Acta Obstetricia et Gynecologica Scandinavica* 81:118–25.

Hirst C 2005 *Rebirthing. Report of the review of maternity services.* Review of maternity services in Queensland, Brisbane.

Ho I, Holroyd E 2002 Chinese women's perceptions of the effectiveness of antenatal education in the preparation for motherhood. *Journal of Advanced Nursing* 38(1):74–85.

Hodnett ED 2000 *Continuity of caregivers for care during pregnancy and childbirth.* Cochrane Database of Systematic Reviews. Issue 1, Art. No. CD000062. DOI: 10.1002/14651858.CD000062.

Hodnett ED, Downe S, Edwards N, Walsh D 2005 *Home-like versus conventional institutional settings for birth (review).* Cochrane Database of Systematic Reviews, Issue 1, Art. No. CD000012.

Holditch-Davis D, Miles M 2000 Mothers' stories about their experiences in the neonatal intensive care unit. *Neonatal Network* 19:13–21.

Homer CSE, Davis GK, Everitt LS 1999 The introduction of a woman-held record into a hospital antenatal clinic: the bring your own records study. *Australian and New Zealand Journal of Obstetrics and Gynaecology* 39(1):54–7.

Jordan S, Emery S, Bradshaw C et al. 2005 The impact of intrapartum analgesia on infant feeding. *BJOG: an International Journal of Obstetrics and Gynaecology* 112(7):927–34.

Kramer MS, Kakuma R 2003 *Optimal duration of exclusive breastfeeding*. Cochrane Review. In Cochrane Library, Issue 1.

Mangesi L, Hofmeyr GJ 2004 *Fetal movement counting for assessment of fetal well-being (protocol)*. Cochrane Database of Systematic Reviews. Issue 3, Art. No. CD004909. DOI: 10.1002/14651858.CD004909.

Medical Records Institute 2006 Continuity of care record (CCR). Available at www.medrecinst.com/pages/about.asp?id=54. Accessed 14 January 2007.

MidCentral Health District Health Board (MCDHB) 2005 *Maternity services strategy*. MCDHB, Palmerston North, New Zealand.

Miles M, Carlson J, Funk S 1996 Sources of support reported by mothers and fathers of infants hospitalized in a neonatal intensive care unit. *Neonatal Network: The Journal of Neonatal Nursing* 15:45–52.

Ministry of Health New Zealand (MOH NZ) 2000 *NZ Public Health and Disability Act 2000*. MOH NZ, Wellington.

Ministry of Health New Zealand (MOH NZ) 2002 *Breastfeeding: a guide to action*. MOH NZ, Wellington. Available at www.moh.govt.nz/.

Ministry of Health New Zealand (MOH NZ) 2006 *Food and nutrition guidelines for healthy pregnant and breastfeeding women. A background paper*. MOH NZ, Wellington.

Moos MK 2003 Preconceptional wellness as a routine objective for women's health care: an integrative strategy. *Journal of Obstetric, Gynecologic, and Neonatal Nursing* 32(4):550–6.

Murray AD, Dolby RM, Nation RL et al. 1981 Effects of epidural anesthesia on newborns and their mothers. *Child Development* 52:71–82.

National Collaborating Centre for Women's and Children's Health 2003 *Antenatal care. Routine care for the healthy pregnant woman. Clinical guideline*. RCOG Press, London. Available at www.rcog.org.uk/resources/Public/pdf/Antenatal_Care.pdf. Accessed 10 January 2007.

National maternity action plan. Available at www.maternitycoalition.org.au/. Accessed 2 August 2006.

Nelson C, Bloom F 1997 Child development and neuroscience. *Child Development* 68(5):970–87.

Nolan ML 1997 Antenatal education—where next? *Journal of Advanced Nursing* 25:1198–204.

Nutbeam D 1998 Health promotion glossary. *Health Promotion International* 13(4):349–64.

Nutbeam D 2000 Health literacy as a public health goal: a challenge for contemporary health education and communication strategies into the 21st century. *Health Promotion International* 15(3):259–67.

Oddy WH, Holt PG, Sly PD et al. 1999 Association between breastfeeding and asthma in 6 year old children: findings of a prospective birth cohort study. *British Medical Journal* 319:815–19.

Parackal SM 2003 *Assessment of risk of foetal alcohol syndrome and other alcohol related effects in New Zealand*. Massey University, Palmerston North, New Zealand.

Pettitt DJ, Forman MR, Hanson RL et al. 1997 Breastfeeding and incidence of non-insulin-dependent diabetes mellitus in Pima Indians. *The Lancet* 350:166–8.

Renkert S, Nutbeam D 2001 Opportunities to improve maternal health literacy through antenatal education: an exploratory study. *Health Promotion International* 16(4):381–8.

Riordan J 1999 Epidurals and breastfeeding. *Breastfeeding Abstracts* 19(2):11–12.

Schore A 2001 Effects of a secure attachment relationship on right brain development, affect regulation, and infant mental health. *Infant Mental Health Journal* 22(1–2):7–66.

Schwarz MK 2005 Parenting preterm infants: a meta-synthesis. *MCN: The American Journal of Maternal/Child Nursing* 30(2):115–20.

Scott JL, Hughes R, Binns C 2001 Factors associated with breastfeeding at discharge and duration of breastfeeding. *Journal of Paediatrics and Child Health* 37(3):254–61.

Spencer N 2000 Social gradients in child health: why do they occur and what can paediatricians do about them? *Ambulatory Child Health* 6:191–202.

Tessier R, Cristo M, Velez S et al. 1998 Kangaroo mother care and the bonding hypothesis. *Pediatrics* 102(2):17–24.

Tew M 1990 *Safer childbirth? A critical history of maternity care*. Chapman & Hall, London.

Torvaldsen S, Roberts CL, Simpson JM et al. 2006 Intrapartum epidural analgesia and breastfeeding: a prospective cohort study. *International Breastfeeding Journal* 1: 24–31.

Truffert P, Goujard J, Dehan M et al. 1998 Outborn status with a medical neonatal transport service and survival without disability at two years. A population-based cohort survey of newborns of less than 33 weeks of gestation. *European Journal of Obstetrics & Gynecology and Reproductive Biology* 79(1):13–18.

UNICEF/World Health Organization 2006 *Baby friendly hospital initiative, revised, updated and expanded for integrated care*, Section 1: background and implementation, preliminary version.

Villar J, Ba'aqeel H, Piaggio G et al. 2001 WHO antenatal care randomized trial for the evaluation of a new model of routine antenatal care. *The Lancet* 357:1551–64.

Villar J, Khan-Neelofur D 2001 Patterns of routine antenatal care for low-risk pregnancy. Cochrane Database of Systematic Reviews, Issue 4, Art. No. CD000934.

von Kries R, Koletzko B, Sauerwald T et al. 1999 Breastfeeding and obesity. *British Medical Journal* 319:147–50.

Waldenstrom U, Nilsson CA 1997 A randomised controlled study of birth center care versus standard maternity care: effects on maternity care. *Birth* 24:17–26.

Whitfield M 2003 Psychosocial effects of intensive care on infants and families after discharge. *Seminars in Neonatology* 8:185–93.

World Health Organization (WHO) 2004 *The importance of caregiver–child interactions for the survival and healthy development of children. A review*. Department of Child and Adolescent Health and Development, WHO, Geneva.

World Health Organization (WHO) 2005 *What is the effectiveness of antenatal care?* (Supplement). WHO, Geneva. Available at www.euro.who.int/document/E87997.pdf. Accessed 4 August 2006.

Chapter 7

Infants and their families

Jennifer Rowe and Margaret Barnes

Learning outcomes

Reading this chapter will help you to:

» define support and apply the concept to nursing support for early parenting

» critique early parenting support programs

» distinguish between universal and targeted health screening and surveillance services

» identify safe, supportive and health promoting practices related to infant feeding

» identify safe, supportive and health promoting practices related to infant settling and sleep

» understand the interactions among sociological, epidemiological and health promotion underpinnings of childhood immunisation

» locate nursing practice and programs in contemporary health service planning and delivery

» identify the knowledge, skills and processes necessary to engage in effective and nursing-proactive practice with families with infants

» critique the organisational role in facilitating responsive nursing-led services, and

» locate sources of population, policy and service information regarding family and child health, provided by government agencies in Australia and New Zealand.

Introduction

Infancy is both an exciting and a challenging time for families. In transition, as the result of the birth of a new child, families are shaped by the child, just as the child is shaped by the family into which they are born. A range of health services is available to support families during this important time. Nurses are at the frontline working in a range of government and private sector services, in institutions and community facilities. Service focus is predominantly on promoting good health for the infant and supporting parenting and families.

In this chapter, some of the challenges that face families during their child's infancy are examined. The reader is provided with a clinical case study that situates the infant and family in the contemporary community. This case is then contextualised and discussed with reference made to central health and psychosocial issues, key nursing practices and innovative programs that are responsive to needs and are informed by current policy. Key topics of interest in nursing families with infants are addressed, including supporting parents, assessing infant growth and development, breastfeeding, settling and sleep, and immunisation.

Setting the scene: a clinical scenario

The nurse

It is 7.30 p.m. and you are the nurse on the 24-hour telephone support service. Frida has just called to talk about her 2-week-old baby girl. She tells you that the baby has been crying for much of the day. Frida says she has tried everything to settle her baby and does not know what else to do. She just does not know how to get through another night alone with her baby.

Frida

Imagine yourself as a late thirties woman, living in a major city, employed in a professional appointment. You have been on leave for just over 5 weeks, having left work 3 weeks prior to the birth of your baby girl, who is now 2 weeks old. You live alone, having split from your long-term partner 12 months ago because he did not want to have children. Following a private arrangement with a sperm donor, you fell pregnant and had a healthy term pregnancy and gave birth at the local hospital assisted by a girlfriend. You went home with your baby 2 days after her birth. You had read voraciously during your pregnancy, mostly about the birth, but also, later in the pregnancy, about breastfeeding and what to expect from the baby in the first year. You had attended five antenatal classes at the hospital. Your baby has been breastfeeding and you feel that you have mastered this skill quite well so far. The baby sleeps next to you in your bed.

This clinical scenario provides a starting point to consider the many healthcare needs of families during the first year of a child's life. It is chosen in part because it helps to disrupt the traditional assumptions of the nuclear family and to draw attention to trends in childbirth and family. Embedded in this scenario are not only specific situational needs, but also universal issues, responses to which are central to the provision of effective family-centred nursing practice.

Families with young children: characteristics in Australia and New Zealand

Frida is one of many women who are having their first baby in their thirties, some of whom are managing alone for any number of reasons. Frida's situation represents a growing family type—the one-parent family with dependent children. Chapter 1 provides a detailed description of the shape of contemporary families in Australia and New Zealand. To reiterate, one-parent families have stabilised in Australia at around 22% of families with dependent children (Australian Bureau of Statistics 2004), while in New Zealand the proportion is still increasing and most recently constituted 18% (Statistics New Zealand 2006).

Frida's decision to go it alone makes her vulnerable, at least financially. The average income of one-parent families is less than that of couple families and a much greater proportion of lone parents receive a government pension (in Australia, 58% compared to 8% of couple families). Lone mothers earn less than lone fathers.

It is important to keep in mind that the single-family household (rather than extended family) is the dominant social grouping in Australian and New Zealand society. Thus, most mothers, whether alone or part of a couple, will experience some degree of isolation as they engage in parenting their young babies. They may find themselves isolated from family and friends at a time when social support is most needed. As parents, they need support so that they are able to find the balance between self and other—that is, to manage their own desires and needs while also providing nurturing care (Rowe 2003) that provides infants with continuity and stability, within a dynamic process of relatedness (Bowden 1997).

Supporting parents and families

Supporting parents in the first months of their new baby's life is a significant practice responsibility for health professionals. This need reflects societal trends where extended family is a minority grouping, and where, for decades, childrearing has been relegated to the invisible space of the domestic frontier, while at the same time, perhaps ironically, subjected to increasing public sector scrutiny and surveillance.

What is support?

Support is an essential aspect of strengths-based and family-centred practice. One of the fundamental tenets of these approaches is to enable families to make informed decisions and choose actions that are informed about things that matter to them (Department of Human Services 2004b). Accepting this assumption is important to the development of services that support families.

Support is conceptualised in different ways in nursing and social science disciplines. Three types appear frequently: informational, tangible or instrumental, and emotional (Heath 2004). Informational support has two important characteristics: accuracy and relevance (House 1981). Emotional support is a complex set of interactions, focused on supporting a person's sense of self or value (Heath 2004, House 1981), or alleviating emotional responses to stressors (Finfgeld-

Connett 2005). Tangible or instrumental support includes a wide range of concrete actions—those providing goods and services (Finfgeld-Connett 2005).

An important aspect of an enabling approach is that regardless of the type, or types, of support appropriate to a situation, the central concern is how parents appraise their situation and define it (Finfgeld-Connett 2005, McCubbin & McCubbin 1993). In addition, it is important to understand the coping styles, strategies and resources used by, or available to, parents.

Supporting parenting on the basis of these assumptions requires more than providing information or educating parents in parentcraft topics. Based on the assumption that parents are the constant in a young child's life negotiating knowledge and experience and needs (Barclay et al. 1997, Rogan et al. 1997, Rowe 2003), it requires practice that places authority in the hands of parents and accepts that parents bring knowledge and are able to be 'the expert'. It infers practising in such a way as to build the capacity of parents to make decisions and, where able, look after their infants, or participate in their infant's care as partners (Rowe & Barnes 2006). The traditional expert (i.e. the nurse as teacher and authority) is thus replaced by a nurse who is an expert in a number of other practices, including helping parents to:

» identify and frame their needs and also their strengths
» reframe their situations, and
» access and utilise a range of resources and thus increase adjustment to parenting (e.g. personal/family community resources).

Priorities for early parenting support

These underpinnings can be applied to supporting early parenting. Some common stressors or challenges have been extensively investigated for men and women, as they negotiate the changing demands, needs, priorities and relationships associated with parenting. Parenting is theorised to involve challenges to both identity and skills in parentcraft or caregiving. These challenges, interweaving ones, may give rise to a range of needs and stressors for both mothers and fathers. Thus, for women, skill in practical caregiving such as breastfeeding and settling an infant can affirm and confirm a maternal role and a narrative of self as mother.

Like women, the transition for men to fatherhood is ongoing and dynamic. The dynamics are similarly complex and involve negotiation and renegotiation of the ideals and realities of care, relationships and other work. Men's transition has not received intense scrutiny, and so specific interactions between beliefs, social discourses and personality are less clearly mapped as they relate to fatherhood and fathering (Dowd 2000, Kaila-Behm & Vehviläinen-Julkunen 2000). For both men and women, successful parenting, marked by acceptance of self and confidence in caregiving, is a keystone in family adjustment and thus family strength.

Programs to support parenting

In both Australia and New Zealand there is a long history of community child health services, reaching out to large proportions of families with babies and young children. Today such services continue to play a role in promoting health and wellbeing for infants and young children, and now incorporate parenting programs to support parents during early childrearing (Barnes et al. 2003, Rowe & Barnes 2006). The need to support parents, as a vital key to strengthening families, is constant whether health services focus on universal or targeted population groups. In Australia, state health departments manage the vast majority of services and so a diverse range of services is offered. See Box 7.1 for an example.

The Royal New Zealand Plunket Society (RNZPS), known as Plunket, is the major New Zealand organisation providing community parenting support services. In Australia, between 75% and well over 90% of new mothers engage with community child health services (Comino & Harris 2003, Department of Human Services 2004a). Plunket sees well over 90% of New Zealand's new mothers (Royal New Zealand Plunket Society n.d.). Because of the vulnerability of disadvantaged groups, targeted services are increasing in an effort to minimise longer term health and social problems.

Traditionally, Well Baby clinics were structured around individual consultations, conducted at health centres, between nurse and parent, usually the mother. Three types of programs have emerged in recent decades that provide support for mothers and, to some extent, fathers, in very different ways. The programs are telephone support lines, parent support groups and home-visiting programs.

Box 7.1 Practice highlight: supporting early parenting

The service

The Tresillian Family Care Centres or, more formally, the Royal Society for the Welfare of Mothers and Babies, is an organisation with a long and rich history in providing support to families with young children in Sydney. Its beginnings date back to the early twentieth century. From its first baby health clinics established in inner Sydney at that time, the service has maintained a continual presence, known by professionals and families across generations simply as Tresillian. Today, it provides a range of targeted services staffed by nurses, psychologists, social workers and medical officers.

Programs

Parents can contact a 24-hour telephone help line if they need advice or assurance, or go online to consult with a nurse, as part of the innovative Messenger Mum strategy. Families who may be struggling with parenting or having difficulties can have a home visit or attend a day-stay clinic for some one-on-one support. For women who may not be coping, or are exhausted or depressed, a tertiary residential service is available.

Developing service and practice

Tresillian has strong links with tertiary education providers to enhance the education and professional development of nurses and is active in research, evaluating outcomes and seeking ways of further developing practice that is responsive to targeted populations (see www.cs.nsw.gov.au/tresillian/default.cfm).

Telephone support lines

Recall the scenario at the beginning of the chapter. Frida had picked up the telephone, seeking help. The availability of community and professional support services can be very important for new parents. Telephone support services are used in a wide variety of health settings, and in the context of new parenting are organised by both state government health services and community organisations. Assessment of and support for immediate needs, and referral to other services, are thought to be significant functions of such services, as well as the 24-hour availability (Lattimer et al. 1998, Sheehan & Barclay 1999).

Telephone contact may be able to be used not only as a response mechanism to parent-identified issues, but also as a contact point for preventive intervention at recognised difficult stages in early parenting. For example, for breastfeeding, if there is contact after discharge from maternity services, during the first week, and again at 8–12 weeks, this may be effective in encouraging breastfeeding maintenance (Department of Health and Human Services Tasmania 2005).

While telephone services are helpful, it is important to keep in mind that evaluation of the standards and effect of these services is limited. Those evaluations that are available suggest that appropriate and specific skills and adequate education on the part of the health professional conducting the telephone service are necessary to ensure accuracy of information provided over the telephone (Andrews et al. 2002). The nurse, as a knowledge worker, must be skilled, not only in the practice area but also in the communication skills needed to consult and counsel on the phone. See Chapter 5 for further information on communication and therapeutic relationships. Given these parameters, effective support for Frida is quite possible.

For Frida, ringing for assistance may have been a last resort; she may be in crisis. Because of this possibility, the nurse in this situation needs, first, to assess her degree of distress and, as far as possible, assess the infant's current wellbeing. The nurse needs to establish that Frida is neither at risk herself, nor of placing her infant at risk, and has the capacity at this time to regroup and continue without seeking assistance as a matter of urgency.

Frida's actions indicate that she is aware of community resources available to her, and this may be the first kernel available to the nurse to provide emotional support—that is, to acknowledge her resourcefulness in seeking assistance. With this key, in a situation that is not ideal, there is opportunity for the nurse to provide Frida with informational and emotional support to address her immediate needs, and also to initiate a discussion that focuses on what she is doing well, and help her recognise her resources at hand. It will be important for the nurse to attempt to gain a picture of Frida and her baby. This is achieved by asking Frida to describe her baby, her baby's behaviour, and her caregiving actions. This process may be quite settling for Frida, as it focuses on concrete things in her world, and provides the nurse with information as a basis for supportive feedback and encouragement.

Encouraging exploration of ways to connect with other supports in the community will assist Frida in identifying resources in the longer term. Providing suggestions may be the most appropriate first start when speaking to Frida, but also taking the time to ask about the times when the baby is settled will highlight to Frida that she has managed well previously. Discussing the wide range of 'normal' infant behaviour and providing information about developmental milestones and changes in infant behaviour and infant care requirements, particularly with regard to feeding, settling and awake period interactions, may address Frida's immediate needs. It is important at this time to ensure that Frida is able to access ongoing support through health services, support groups or family.

Parent support groups

Sometimes known as facilitated peer networking (Barnes et al. 2004, Scott et al. 2001), the parenting group takes many forms. It refers to a small group of peers—new parents, usually facilitated by a nurse, at least in the first instance. The immediate advantage is that this service puts parents, most usually mothers, in touch with each other, a process that is increasingly difficult for mothers to do informally via family and friendship networks. Women such as Frida can be put in touch with other women, and young children. See Box 7.2 for an example of a parent support service.

The scene is then set for women to share experiences, knowledge and ideas with each other. This sharing attends to both emotional and informational support needs. Women have a space to share the important stories of caregiving minutiae, relationship and family dynamics, and reflections on the maternal role. From these interactions, women continue negotiating and confirming their role (Börjesson et al. 2004), and testing the information they glean in their own context (Rowe 2003, Rowe & Barnes 2006). In addition, it provides the opportunity for anticipatory guidance on caregiving topics such as breastfeeding, settling and sleep, immunisation and important developmental steps for the infants.

Box 7.2 Practice highlight: Early Bird Program, South East Sydney and Illawarra Area Health Service

This service was established in the late 1990s for parents of babies up to 2 months of age. Based on principles of enabling parents through partnership and peer support, it aims to promote parents' exchange of expertise, and their confidence with decision making, and satisfaction with parenting. Recruiting parents as soon after a baby's birth as possible, the program involves the use of a series of facilitated support group meetings for parents, most usually mothers.

It is anticipated that groups, or some members of groups, will develop ongoing relationships and this is encouraged by the facilitating nurse. It also assumes a partnership between the parent and the facilitating nurse, who brings expertise on a range of topics. Parents continue to have access to individual consultation with nurses if they require it and also for ongoing child health assessment.

Practice development

This program is an interesting example of parenting support groups, and also of principles of practice development. It is nurse-initiated and led, established as a result of a local service review and developed with involvement of nurse/midwifery researchers and clinicians. It includes key structural elements and strategies for clinical nurses to use in its implementation. This has been achieved through the production and wide distribution of a user's manual for nurses, which contains information about running groups, communication strategies, challenges nurse facilitators may face, and proforma and standardised evaluation tools to use with groups. Thus, it equips nurses with the tools they need in a range of settings to implement and evaluate the program. It recognises the need to include education and professional development for clinicians.

With an evaluation mechanism built into the program, ongoing responsiveness in the program is enhanced. Further, evaluation has been more widely disseminated through publication of evaluation data in the peer-reviewed literature (see Kruske et al. 2004).

Evaluations demonstrate the effectiveness of peer support to help parents build confidence and increase breastfeeding maintenance (Kruske et al. 2004). They also generate longer term social networks for parents and families (Scott et al. 2001). One evaluation study found that women appreciated becoming involved in a support program as soon after the birth of their baby as possible (Kruske et al. 2004). Evaluations also raise a debate about whether these are mothering or parenting groups, due to the small involvement of fathers in these initiatives (Scott et al. 2001).

Home-visiting programs

Home visiting is a third type of parenting support program currently receiving significant support in policy and health service strategy. In New Zealand, a universal home-visiting service is offered by Plunket to families with children under 5 years of age, providing both child developmental assessment and parenting support (Royal New Zealand Plunket Society n.d.). It has been used at different times in Australia's history with maternal and child health services. Currently, targeted home visiting is used in a number of Australian states—for example, in Victoria, where up to 15 hours of support can be offered to vulnerable families with a child less than 12 months of age, and who are experiencing parenting difficulties (Department of Human Services 2004a).

Systematic reviews of home-visiting programs in the United States, Canada and the United Kingdom have demonstrated that there are some positive outcomes in the environment, maternal wellbeing and parenting (Gomby et al. 1999, Jack et al. 2005, Kearney et al. 2000, Kendrick et al. 2000). The first Australian research evaluating a home-visiting program for vulnerable families (Armstrong et al. 2000) demonstrated short-term reduction in parental stress, maternal depression and more parent–child interactions in the home-visiting cohort, but no demonstrable maintenance of a positive intervention impact on maternal mood in the 2-year follow up (Fraser et al. 2000). Despite the poor long-term benefits, this program was implemented widely throughout Queensland. The success of the program is challenged by a number of factors, including limited training in maternal psychopathology for the nurses, and concurrent maternal substance abuse problems.

Equivocal results among recent trials show that the specific content of home-visiting programs that induces positive outcome is somewhat illusive, and successes are marginal. The need to critically reappraise the nature and content of programs is thus underscored. There is growing acknowledgment that home-visiting programs need to be clearly targeted and supplemented by psychological treatments adapted for use in the home. Given the above, it is clear research needs to continue, and programs developed in which individual parental factors as well as the social environment are addressed.

The evaluations that are available point to some implications for nurses and health services providing home visitation:

- Home-visiting nurses need to have adequate and advanced competencies and experience in the range of social and health issues that they will address with families (Fraser et al. 2000, Department of Human Services 2004a, Kearney et al. 2000).
- Support for staff in terms of supervision and ongoing training and development is also recognised as a key ingredient for effective practice (Armstrong et al. 2000, Department of Human Services 2004b, Gomby et al. 1999).

- It has been theorised that it is the relationship between visitor and parent that is central to positive outcomes (Jack et al. 2005, Ammerman et al. 2006).
- In home-visiting situations, acceptance by the mother and family and the development of a respectful relationship, and sense of mutuality between visitor and mother, will be key requirements (Jack et al. 2005).

Thus, this service requires effective assessment and targeting, experienced and specifically educated and trained staff, and active organisational support (Kemp et al. 2005). Family-centred practice rather than system-centred practice requires that the maternal and child health nurse practise as a facilitator. Nurses must be well prepared, have a good knowledge base of risks and protective factors that influence parenting and family adjustment, and must have the skills to work with parents so that they might build on existing strengths and their personal, family and other resources (Department of Human Services 2004b).

Assessing and promoting infant health and wellbeing

Supporting Frida is one service nurses can provide. Additionally, there is potential for them to support the growth and development of her infant daughter in a range of preventive health assessment and screening practices, and interventions.

Health screening and surveillance

For parents, knowing that a baby is well and progressing along the established norms is often affirmed in data they gather from child health nurses and document in personal health records. Frida and indeed all families will leave maternity services with their newborn and a personal health record for their child. In this record, among other things, specific physical, cognitive and motor skills milestones can be mapped out, potential health problems and symptoms to watch for identified, and schedules for assessment of the child's development and immunisation set out.

The personal health record is treated as both a data archive and health education tool. Potentially, it provides a history of the child. In both Australia and New Zealand, parents can use this record and then access professionals to conduct the appropriate assessment—in child health clinics, general practice rooms and pharmacies, to name a few. See Box 7.3, which highlights the development of growth charts, a central feature of the personal health records. An evaluation of the use of personal records by parents in the United Kingdom revealed that the personal health records functioned best as records and least well as health education tools (Wright & Reynolds 2006). This evaluation study also found that a more comprehensive education book given to all parents of newborns was also poorly used. Further data on the use of the record is needed in Australia and New Zealand.

As can be seen from the above discussion of parenting support, child assessment can be conducted in a range of settings and contexts. Health screening and surveillance have been promoted in both Australia and New Zealand over a long period of time. Child growth standards are widely used as a tool in public health, medicine and by government and health organisations for monitoring the wellbeing of children and for detecting children or populations who are not growing properly

Box 7.3 Practice highlight: tracking growth

So many babies have had their height and weight tracked through infancy and recorded on growth charts. This practice started in the late nineteenth century and continues to the present day. Charts used through the last decades of the twentieth century were based on norms for children from 1929–75 who were predominantly American middle-class and bottle-fed (Centers for Disease Control and Prevention 2000). The Centers for Disease Control and Prevention (CDC) in the United States produced more discerning charts in 2000, which are based on norms from both bottle-fed and breastfed infants. These have been widely used. More recently, the World Health Organization (WHO) produced new charts as a single reference point, also establishing breastfed infants as the normative model for growth and development (2007). Information about the WHO child growth standards, their development, as well as the charts, can be accessed on the WHO webpage.

It is interesting to examine these changes, and reflect on the changing social practices and the implications of these for establishing norms for child growth and development and, inevitably, parenting activities. Further, the changes reflect the interaction of epidemiology, science and health policy over time. What does not change is the fact that formula and breastfed infants have different patterns of growth in the first few months of life. Breastfed infants tend to grow more rapidly than formula-fed infants in the first 2 months of life and then more slowly in comparison during the third and fourth months.

Implications for nursing practice

It is important that measures such as these are used as reference points, not standards to be met. Measuring growth must be conducted within the context of a health promoting framework, not an isolated test for babies, and their parents, to pass or fail.

Reader activity

The CDC website at www.cdc.gov/growthcharts/ and the WHO website provide comprehensive information on the charts, their use and the basis for changes. Readers are encouraged to spend some time examining this information.

or who are underweight or overweight and may require specific medical or public health responses. Regular assessment of a baby's growth and developmental progress through infancy and the early years of life continues, often under the umbrella term 'weighing and measuring'. It is not the intention in this chapter to describe those assessment activities, but rather to provide readers with a more critical lens in order that they have the opportunity to consider a future-focused practice.

In Australia, in 2002, a review of evidence for child health surveillance and screening (National Health and Medical Research Council 2002) marked a turning point in the focus and thinking about these practices. The executive summary of the review is worth quoting as it brings into stark relief the issues and challenges facing policy makers, service planners, researchers and clinicians in this arena (p. 2):

> 'There is surprisingly little evidence for the effectiveness of screening programs in many domains (that is not to say the corollary is true—for some, there is inadequate evidence for lack of effectiveness either). There are scant data about

> cost effectiveness. There are major issues of program quality, monitoring of compliance with referrals for assessment, and whether facilities exist in many communities for assessment and follow up. There are concerns that much attention is paid to the test or procedure itself and little to the main elements of a community-wide program. In some cases, there is little evidence that therapy alters outcomes.'

The review does not attempt to deter the intent of early detection; indeed, it encourages this agenda together with early intervention. It argues the need for services that are based on evidence. Importantly, the review highlighted that where there is sufficient evidence for screening and surveillance activities, these are only useful if conducted within a program or system. That is to say that conducting an isolated test that the infant either passes or fails is not an effective preventive strategy. What is required is a system or program that contains clear protocols, well-trained staff, clear referral and guidance pathways, and standardised procedures for ongoing follow-up, as well as clear documentation (National Health and Medical Research Council 2002, Child and Youth Health Intergovernmental Partnership 2002).

Two service directions are becoming commonplace in the face of evidence:

1. universal, and
2. targeted.

What is clear is that responsiveness to family-specific situations and needs is important, rather than the more traditional one-size-fits-all approach. Further, programs are needed that account for child, parent, family and life events, as well as broader social or community factors.

These tensions and concerns extend to the value of a range of activities designed to prevent ill health and promote good health. This knowledge has implications for nurses and the programs that are offered to families during the first year of a child's life. For example, there is good evidence that activities to promote breastfeeding, infant sleep conditions and immunisation are effective.

Breastfeeding

Frida tells the nurse on the telephone that she feels breastfeeding has been going well. With a baby 2 weeks old, this is a good thing. Frida, over 30, and with a high level of education, is representative of the largest age group of women likely to start and continue breastfeeding.

The World Health Organization (2003) recommends exclusive breastfeeding of infants until they are 6 months old and continued breastfeeding with other foods until they are 2 years of age. However, in Australia, only 54% of babies continue to be exclusively breastfed in the first 3 months and very few at 6 months (Australian Bureau of Statistics 2003). These figures are reflective of the New Zealand situation with less breastfeeding maintenance in Maori and other non-European populations (Ministry of Health New Zealand 2002). See Chapter 6 for further information about breastfeeding initiation.

There are a number of barriers to maintaining high breastfeeding rates. The societal influences are complex. However, health service issues, particularly as they affect the quality and continuity of care, also influence breastfeeding practices (Ministry of Health New Zealand 2002). Antenatal, perinatal and early child health services all have an important part to play in encouraging good infant feeding practices. There are a number of requisites for services:

» Services need to be adequately resourced, be accessible and offer appropriately targeted services, with appropriately skilled staff.
» Services must be able to link parents with other parents and families, and with a range of support and intervention services (e.g. the Australian Breastfeeding Association or lactation consultants).
» Services must network rather than act as silos in order to promote health and wellbeing. See Chapter 2 for information about silo culture in healthcare and program development.

In Frida's situation, learning about her intentions and knowledge about breastfeeding will be important to support her continued practice. Breastfeeding practice and soothing/settling are also linked with each other. Daily use of a pacifier in the first month, for example, is linked with a decrease in breastfeeding. Thus, the nurse needs to have a good understanding of breastfeeding and also settling and infant sleep.

Settling and infant sleep

Sleep and settling are immediate concerns for Frida. In the previous 200 years, infant settling and sleep practices in families in western countries have diverged greatly from the practices of history and the majority of the world's population (McKenna et al. 1993, McKenna & Joyce n.d.). Today, in countries such as Australia and New Zealand, not all parents will consider doing what Frida does—that is, bedshare with an infant. In fact, many will be fearful about doing so. Some will keep their young infants in a crib or cot close to their own bed. Others prefer their infants to sleep alone, believing that co-sleeping practices make the child dependent or spoil the child, or that the child will never sleep alone, or that this is the only way they will get sufficient sleep themselves. Many believe (and most certainly desire) that an infant of 3 months and older is capable of safely sleeping alone, and through the night.

Whatever the position, settling a baby and getting a baby to sleep is a significant issue in the day-to-day lives of parents, and one that reflects very clearly their personal negotiation into parenting (Rowe 2003). Responding to this need becomes integral to child health nursing programs. In addition, promoting safe practices is important as a universal health service, both to promote health and minimise risk.

A large amount of public health attention is focused on safe infant sleep practices, largely because of Sudden Infant Death Syndrome (now classified as unexplained unexpected death in infancy as distinct from explained unexpected infant deaths), a baffling and devastating event which until the mid-1990s claimed the lives of more infants than any other cause, about 2–4 in 1000. The 1990s saw a significant downturn in this statistic, with an 84% reduction cited following the introduction of a public campaign (SIDS and KIDS 2005). (During this time, further classification and definition of SIDS deaths and clarification of autopsy procedures has occurred, which is also likely to influence the statistics.)

The premise of the campaign is that a safe sleeping arrangement for infants is for them to be positioned on their backs, without bumpers or other loose bedding or soft toys, in a smoke-free environment. It is recommended that cots are placed in parents' bedrooms for night-time sleeping as a protective mechanism. This represents a form of co-sleeping. Box 7.4 clarifies the differences between co-sleeping and bedsharing.

Box 7.4 Practice highlight: distinguishing between co-sleeping and bedsharing

It is important to have a clear understanding of the distinction between these two terms. Co-sleeping can include arrangements where the child is in close proximity to the parents on a shared or separate sleeping surface (e.g. a cot beside the bed or a three-sided cot flush against the bed). Bedsharing refers specifically to arrangements in which the infant sleeps in the same bed as the parents. The room needs to be smoke-free.

Bedsharing is only recommended when the surface is firm without loose or too much bedding, poor ventilation in the room, or where there is risk of the infant becoming stuck between mattress and frame, or of falling out, and, importantly, where parents are not affected by alcohol, prescription or illicit drugs. If any of these conditions are present in the sleep environment, a co-sleeping arrangement with the infant close but on a separate surface is preferable (McKenna & Joyce n.d., SIDS and KIDS 2005).

Nursing practice promoting safe family sleep environments

The challenges for nurses working with families to help them meet the demands they face is not to increase their fears, but rather to provide them with options that are protective, health promoting and nurturing for the infant. Options need to help parents to create realistic and safe sleeping environments for their infant and themselves, according to their specific physical environment and lifestyle needs. To do this, nurses need to first interrogate their own values and ensure that they are guided by evidence and family-centred principles. Evidence suggests that:

- There is nothing to be gained by an infant sleeping in a solitary place, away from the company of others (McKenna & Joyce n.d.).
- There are some sleep environmental conditions, such as a smoke-free room and use of a firm mattress, either bed or cot, and certain bedclothes, that promote safety (SIDS & KIDS 2005).
- Back sleeping is a safe position for infants (SIDS & KIDS 2005).

This and other evidence needs to be incorporated within an individualised, dynamic and negotiated process in which parents are supported to make their own decisions.

To do this, nurses also need to understand how parents appraise their situation. For example, what are parents' assumptions about normal sleep for infants and their own sleep expectations? Nurses need to assess parents' understanding of their babies' behaviours, and how they interpret what their infants are signalling, in order to help them increase their knowledge, where this is needed. Nurses need to help them negotiate their options. For example, is there room in the parents' bedroom for a cot for an infant up to 12 months of age? Are there settling strategies they can try? Are there other family or friends who can help, and when and what might they do?

Immunisation

The third health promotion area to consider is immunisation. It is beyond the scope of this chapter to provide a detailed analysis of the historical debates and clinical practice guidelines and issues that have surrounded childhood immunisation. Rather, it is the intention here to refer the reader to appropriate information regarding childhood immunisation schedules and to challenge readers to consider and inform themselves about important practice and service factors.

Childhood immunisation coverage rates are measured in Australia at 1, 2 and 6 years. In 2006, they were reported as 90.8%, 92.2% and 86.2%, respectively (Australian Government Medicare n.d.). In New Zealand, the rate in 2005 at 2 years was 77% (Ministry of Health New Zealand 2006). The standard schedule and vaccines vary in each country, but can be easily accessed via the immunisation handbooks for each country, available online.

Immunisation can be provided by a range of health professionals in a range of settings, including general practitioners, hospitals and community health services. Each nurse providing immunisations as part of their clinical practice needs to consider a number of things if they are to promote best practice. We suggest that readers access the handbooks for immunisation for both Australia and New Zealand. For information on New Zealand childhood immunisation, go to:

» Ministry of Health New Zealand (MOH NZ) 2006. *Immunisation handbook 2006*. MOH NZ, Wellington. Available at www.moh.govt.nz.

For information on Australian childhood immunisation, go to:

» Department of Health and Ageing at www9.health.gov.au/immhandbook/.

Use this information to respond to each of the following questions:

1. What diseases is population immunisation combating? How are these diseases transmitted?
2. What is the current immunisation schedule?
3. What are the commonly used vaccine preparations?
4. What is current best practice for vaccine administration?
5. What is current best practice for vaccine storage and transport?
6. What are the adverse effects of immunisations? (The *Australian immunisation handbook*, available on the Department of Health and Ageing website at http://www9.health.gov.au/immhandbook/, provides a useful table identifying disease, method of transmission, effects of disease in type and rate, and adverse effects of immunisation in type and rate.)
7. What clinical conditions may delay or contraindicate immunisation?
8. What are the registration and recording procedures for childhood immunisation?

Nurses also need to consider past and present immunisation debates and the issues these raise for parents—in other words, knowing what the talk on the street is. Informed consent is an important aspect of the immunisation procedure, as it is for other medical treatments. See Chapter 4 for a full discussion of informed consent in treatment and research.

Parents need to have clear and correct information, not only about the vaccine but also about the disease and its adverse effects. They must also be able to interpret their personal experiences as part of their decision making. They have a right to accurate information, provided in a climate of respect for their experience. Resources are available to assist health professionals understand parent concerns and to respond to them. See, for example, the National Centre for Immunisation Research (NCIRS) at www.ncirs.usyd.edu.au/facts/resources_patient-parent%20concern%20about%20immunisation.pdf.

As advocates and change agents, nurses are responsible for individual practice and for health service development. Thus, nurses need to consider the service they work in with regard to immunisation practice:

1. Are current resources for health professionals available to staff?
2. Is appropriate professional development available and valued?
3. Are resources to assist parent/carer knowledge about immunisation available and accessible?

Conclusion

In this chapter, a number of nursing-led services and programs that support families with young infants were introduced. We focused on the provision of parenting support, and the assessment of infant growth and development. In addition, we looked at three important and at times controversial topics in early childrearing and child health: infant feeding, infant settling and sleep, and immunisation. Throughout the discussion, the relevance of nursing practice to the lives and health of families with infants has been demonstrated.

A changed role from the traditional one is argued, in which the expertise of the nurse is in facilitation, applying expert knowledge to help families make decisions about caregiving practices for their infants and also to support parents as they face the significant challenges parenthood brings to everyday life and to their understanding of the needs, priorities and desires of their lives.

Practice tips

» *Start early*: women are challenged in the first few days after taking their newborn babies home.
» *Do less*: nurses need to be less the expert teacher advisor and more the expert facilitator to promote parent expertise, wisdom and confidence.
» *Prepare clinicians* with skills and the tools to implement programs and to assess health and wellbeing.
» *Skill nurses* to practise in culturally safe and competent ways.
» *Build* on existing individual and family strengths.
» *Support families* to appraise their situation, identify their needs, determine their options and make decisions that will work for them.
» *Provide* clear and standardised protocols, including sufficient guidance and detail to be used by clinicians.

» *Apply* evidence in interactive processes with parents, not prescriptions.
» *Participate* in service development as change agents, advocates and integral members of multidisciplinary healthcare teams.

Useful resources

There are many websites that provide useful information and also give you insight into what is happening at policy and service planning level in both Australia and New Zealand. It is best to access the federal, state and district or local council websites and search the health sections for information on families, children, and health and wellbeing.

For statistical information about family characteristics and trends:

» Australian Bureau of Statistics (ABS) 2004 *Family characteristics, Australia*. Available at www.abs.gov.au/Austats/abs@.nsf/.
» Statistics New Zealand 2006 *Census data*. Available at www.stats.govt.nz/census/default.htm.

For information on breastfeeding policy/guidelines, support and research:

» www.who.int/topics/breastfeeding/en/
» www.breastfeeding.asn.au/
» www.bfhi.org.au/
» www.babyfriendly.org.nz/
» www.lalecheleague.org.nz/

For information on infant settling and sleep:

» McKenna JJ, Joyce EP n.d. *Mother–baby behavioral sleep laboratory*. Department of Anthropology, University of Notre Dame, Indiana. Available at www.nd.edu/~jmckenn1/lab/index.html.
» SIDS and KIDS 2005 Homepage. Available at www.sidsandkids.org/.

For information on immunisation:

» Department of Health and Ageing: www9.health.gov.au/immhandbook/.
» Ministry of Health New Zealand (MOH NZ) 2006. *Immunisation handbook 2006*. MOH NZ, Wellington. Available at www.moh.govt.nz/moh.nsf/238fd5fb4fd051844c256669006aed57/555b0e9a841bea3ecc2571470017dab1?OpenDocument#intro.

Other useful sites are:

» Royal New Zealand Plunket Society (RNZPS): www.plunket.org.nz/.
» Tresillian Family Care Centres: www.cs.nsw.gov.au/tresillian/default.cfm.

References

Ammerman R, Stevens J, Putnam F et al. 2006 Predictors of early engagement in home visitation. *Journal of Family Violence* 21(2):105–15.

Andrews J, Armstrong K, Fraser F 2002 Professional telephone advice to parents with sick children: time for quality control. *Journal of Paediatric Child Health* 38:23–6.

Armstrong K, Fraser J, Dadds M, Morris J 2000 Promoting secure attachment, maternal mood and child health in a vulnerable population. *Journal of Paediatrics and Child Health* 36:555–62.

Australian Bureau of Statistics (ABS) 2003 *Breastfeeding in Australia 2001*. Available at www.abs.gov.au / AUSSTATS / abs @.nsf/ cat / 4810.0.55.001.

Australian Bureau of Statistics (ABS) 2004 *Family characteristics, Australia*. Available at www.abs.gov.au / Austats / abs@.nsf/ .

Australian Government Medicare n.d. Available at www.medicareaustralia.gov.au/ providers / health_statistics / statistical_reporting / acir.htm.

Barclay L, Everitt L, Rogan F et al. 1997 Becoming a mother: an analysis of women's experience of early motherhood. *Journal of Advanced Nursing* 25(4):719–28.

Barnes M, Courtney M, Pratt J, Walsh A 2003 Contemporary child health nursing practice: services provided and challenges faced in metropolitan and outer Brisbane areas. *Collegian* 10(4):14–19.

Barnes M, Courtney M, Pratt, J, Walsh A 2004 The roles, responsibilities and professional development needs of child health nurses. *Focus on Health Professional Education* 6(1):52–63.

Börjesson B, Paperin C, Lindell M 2004 Maternal support during the first year of infancy. *Journal of Advanced Nursing* 45(6):588–94.

Bowden P 1997 *Caring. A gender sensitive ethics*. Routledge, London.

Centers for Disease Control and Prevention (CDC), Department of Health and Human Services, United States 2000 *CDC growth charts: USA*. Available at www.cdc.gov / growthcharts / . Last revised April 2005.

Child and Youth Health Intergovernmental Partnership (CHIP) 2002 *Child health screening and surveillance: supplementary document: context and next steps*. Available at www.nhmrc.gov.au / publications.

Comino E, Harris E 2003 Maternal and infant services: examination of access in a culturally diverse community. *Journal of Paediatric Child Health* 39:95–9.

Department of Health and Human Services Tasmania (FCYHS) 2005 *Strategic plan for early childhood 2005–2008*. Available at www.dhhs.tas.gov.au.

Department of Human Services (DHS) 2004a *BestStart*. Available at www.beststart. vic.gov.au.

Department of Human Services (DHS) 2004b *Future directions for the Victorian Maternal and Child Health Service, State of Victoria*. Available at www.office-for-children.vic.gov.au / ecs / library / publications / mch / future_directions.

Dowd N 2000 *Redefining fatherhood*. New York University Press, New York.

Finfgeld-Connett D 2005 Clarification of social support. *Journal of Nursing Scholarship* 37(1):4–9.

Fraser J, Armstrong K, Morris J, Dadds M 2000 Home visiting intervention for vulnerable families with newborns: follow up results of a randomised controlled trial. *Child Abuse and Neglect* 24(11):399–1429.

Gomby S, Culross P, Behrman R 1999 Home visiting: recent program evaluations—analysis and recommendations. *The Future of Children* 9(1):4–26.

Government of South Australia Child, Youth and Women's Services. Child and Youth Health website: www.cyh.com / Default.aspx?p=1.

Heath H 2004 Assessing and delivering parent support. In M Hoghughi & N Long (eds), *Handbook of parenting. Theory and research for practice*. Sage, London, pp. 311–33.

House J 1981 *Work stress and social support.* Addison-Wesley, Reading, Massachusetts.

Jack S, DiCenso A, Lohfeld, L 2005 A theory of maternal engagement with public health nurses and family visitors. *Journal of Advanced Nursing* 49(2):182–90.

Kaila-Behm A, Vehviläinen-Julkunen K 2000 Ways of being a father: how first-time fathers and public health nurses perceive men as fathers. *International Journal of Nursing Studies* 37:199–205.

Kearney M, York R, Deatrick J 2000 Effects of home visits to vulnerable young families. *Journal of Nursing Scholarship* 32(4):369–76.

Kemp L, Anderson T, Travaglia J, Harris E 2005 Sustained nurse home visiting in early childhood: exploring Australian nursing competencies. *Public Health Nursing* 22(3):54–259.

Kendrick D, Elkan R, Hewitt M et al. 2000 Does home visiting improve parenting and the quality of the home environment? A systematic review and meta analysis. *Archives of Diseases of Childhood* 82:443–51.

Kruske S, Schmied V, Sutton I, O'Hare J 2004 Mothers' experiences of facilitated peer support groups and individual child health nursing support: a comparative evaluation. *Journal of Perinatal Education* 13(3):31–8.

Lattimer V, George S, Thompson F et al. (South Wiltshire Out of Hours Project Group) 1998 Safety and effectiveness of nurse telephone consultations in out of hours primary care: a randomised controlled trial. *British Medical Journal* 317:1054–9.

McCubbin M, McCubbin H 1993 Families coping with illness: the resiliency model of family stress, adjustment, and adaptation. In C Danielson, B Hamel-Bissell & P Winstead-Fry (eds), *Families, health, and illness.* Mosby, St Louis, Missouri, pp. 21–63.

McKenna JJ, Joyce EP n.d. *Mother–baby behavioral sleep laboratory.* Department of Anthropology, University of Notre Dame, Indiana. Available at www.nd.edu/~jmckenn1/lab/index.html.

McKenna JJ, Thoman E, Anders T et al. 1993 Infant–parent co-sleeping in an evolutionary perspective: implications for understanding infant sleep development and the sudden infant death syndrome. *Sleep* 16(3):263–82.

Ministry of Health New Zealand (MOH NZ) 2002 *Breastfeeding: a guide to action.* MOH NZ, Wellington. Available at www.moh.govt.nz/.

Ministry of Health New Zealand (MOH NZ) 2006 *Immunisation handbook 2006.* MOH NZ, Wellington. Available at www.moh.govt.nz/moh.nsf/238fd5fb4fd051844c256669006aed57/555b0e9a841bea3ecc2571470017dab1?OpenDocument#intro.

National Health and Medical Research Council (NHMRC) 2002 *Child health surveillance and screening: a critical review of the evidence.* Available at http://nhmrc.gov.au/publications/.

Rogan F, Schmied V, Barclay L et al. 1997 'Becoming a mother': developing a new theory of early motherhood. *Journal of Advanced Nursing* 25(5):877–85.

Rowe J 2003 A room of their own: the social landscape of infant sleep. *Nursing Inquiry* 10(3):184–92.

Rowe J, Barnes M 2006 The role of child health nurses in enhancing mothering know-how. *Collegian* 13(4):22–6.

Royal New Zealand Plunket Society (RNZPS) n.d. Plunket on-line. Available at www.plunket.org.nz/.

Scott D, Brady S, Glynn P 2001 New mother groups as a social network intervention: consumer and maternal and child health nurse perspectives. *Australian Journal of Advanced Nursing* 18(4):23–9.

Sheehan A, Barclay L 1999 *An audit of 24-hour parent help lines across Australia*. Good Beginnings Project. Available at www.goodbeginnings.net.au/main.php?page=library/.

SIDS and KIDS 2005 Homepage. Available at www.sidsandkids.org/.

Statistics New Zealand 2006 *Census data*. Available at www.stats.govt.nz/census/default.htm.

World Health Organization (WHO) 2003 *Global strategy for infant and young child feeding*. WHO, Geneva. Available at www.who.int/nutrition/publications/infantfeeding/en/index.html.

World Health Organization (WHO) 2007 WHO child growth standards. WHO Geneva. Available at www.who.int/childgrowth/standards/en/index.html.

Wright C, Reynolds L 2006 How widely are personal child health records used and are they effective health education tools? A comparison of two records. *Child Care, Health and Development* 32(1):55–61.

Chapter 8

Early childhood: health promotion and acute illness episodes

Catherine Maginnis and Linda Shields[1]

Learning outcomes

Reading this chapter will help you to:

- understand the influence of the school and childcare environment on children's health and wellbeing
- define a Health Promoting School
- appreciate the role of nurses in the school health promoting environment
- identify key health issues in early childhood
- identify common acute illnesses
- discuss contexts of care for the acutely ill child
- understand children's and parents' needs when a child is hospitalised
- contextualise and critique family-centred care, and
- develop an understanding of principles of nursing practice that strengthens the health and wellbeing of young children and their families.

Introduction

Early childhood is a time of development, play and exploration—a time when childcare, preschool or school are an important part of life. It is a time that is often

1 We would like to acknowledge the contribution of Margaret Barnes and Jennifer Rowe to the preparation of the final version of this chapter.

trouble free, but also a time where healthy school environments and family support may be strengthening and assist the development of healthy patterns of behaviour and meaningful relationships. It is also a time punctuated by episodes of acute illness, recurrent infections and injury. During these episodes, parents will be the primary care providers, interacting with health professionals in a range of settings in order to facilitate their child's recovery and health.

In this chapter, the reader is provided with an overview of the young child's capacities, interests and social environment. Major sources of influence and support are set out, particularly as these may facilitate young children's health and wellbeing. Health promoting activities are discussed, as these can be integrated in both school and health services. Sources of acute illness are identified and the contexts for treatment and care for young children with an acute illness episode are discussed.

Early childhood: the play and school years

Early childhood can be defined as the stage of steady but slow growth and development between toddlerhood and puberty. This life stage focuses on 'play, body mastery and skill development' (Oates et al. 2001 p. 6). Early development of preschool-aged children is characterised by lots of activity and discovery. Motor skills advance and language and social relationships develop. As young children increasingly develop a self-concept, they have increasing independence (Wong et al. 2006). During middle childhood, children broaden their social relationships and begin to further develop competency in all areas (Wong et al. 2006).

For preschoolers, major milestones include development of gross motor skills—for example, walking up and down steps, skipping and hopping, learning to balance on one leg, and to ride a tricycle or bike with training wheels. Fine motor skills include building towers with cubes, drawing and copying shapes, beginning to use scissors and learning to tie shoe laces (although the age of Velcro is making this last activity redundant as a means of demonstrating developmental competence).

It is a time when vocabulary increases, as does the ability to construct sentences. Young children can recount recent events and state their name and address. They may count up to 20 or more and know and can sing nursery rhymes. By age 5 they like jokes and riddles. They enjoy being read to and ask lots of questions. They have the potential to develop and use an extensive vocabulary, have good comprehension of spoken language and can narrate stories themselves (Sheridan 1994, Wong et al. 2006). See Box 8.1 for details of a reading program aimed at this particular age group.

Preschoolers like to help parents and caregivers with chores and engage actively in play. They try to abide by rules and please others and are mostly independent in self-care activities. For securely attached young children living in supportive environments, interaction with families goes from rebelling, frustrated and argumentative, to getting on well with parents and seeking them out for reassurance and security, especially when starting preschool and school (Sheridan 1994, Wong et al. 2006).

These abilities continue to develop in primary-school-aged children, as they become more independent. Play becomes more focused on physical skills, intellectual ability and fantasy. Rituals and conforming become a major focus in this age group. Team play emerges and peer interaction with rules, referees

Box 8.1 Practice highlight: the Let's Read Program

The Let's Read Program is run by the Royal Children's Hospital Melbourne's Centre for Community Child Health. Designed as a sustainable community-based program, it facilitates early child health and development through promoting reading in the 4–6 months to 5-year age group, particularly in disadvantaged groups. The rationale for the program is the important research evidence linking brain development and language and literacy skill development, and also the ongoing relationship between literacy, life chances and self-esteem. The program has two components:

1. training key community-based professionals such as child health nurses, and
2. providing resource materials, including reading guidelines and books for community-based groups.

Read about it on the website at www.rch.org.au/ccch/research/index.cfm?doc_id=5821#about.

Questions

1. Look at the risk and protective factors table in Chapter 1 (Table 1.1). How does a program like this interact with this balance of risk and protective factors in ways that might strengthen a child's wellbeing and future?
2. Have you ever thought that helping improve language and emergent literacy for young children could be a major health promoting role for you to undertake?
3. More generally, how could you use reading and picture books with children and their families in health promoting activities?

Perhaps you could build an archive of useful titles. Don't forget that appropriate, accessible and affordable are key elements to consider.

and playing other teams. This helps stimulate growth, as they must learn rules, make judgments, plan strategies, and assess weaknesses and strengths of their own team and the opposition. It is a high-activity age; but children at this stage also enjoy quiet and solitude. Self-concept and body image begin to be influenced by peers, but positive experiences can be promoted by family and other adults or organisations. This gives children a feeling of success and more confidence about themselves. A positive self-concept leads to self-respect and confidence (Wong et al. 2006).

Setting the scene: promoting health in young children

Gary, a community nurse, is approached by the principal of the local primary school to assist in planning a 'Health Expo'. The Expo is based on the Health Promoting Schools model and is going to be a major community event this year. In your area, nurses have not been active in school-aged screening or health promotion, so you welcome the invitation. The planning group discusses involving the two local childcare centres as well, and have invited parents to join the group.

The school and childcare environment as sites for health promotion

Schools and childcare environments are considered appropriate settings for strategic implementation of health promotion programs that will facilitate health-enhancing environments (Hayden 2002b). Children spend a large part of their day in environments other than the home, so it is important that these environments are health promoting.

Childcare

Many young children attend some form of formal or informal childcare on a regular basis. The use of these facilities is increasing with changes in working patterns of parents, an increase in single-parent families and high mobility rates where families are separated from extended family support (Australian Institute of Health and Welfare 2007a). The most common reason cited for using childcare is work related for before/after school care, family daycare and long daycare (Australian Bureau of Statistics 2005). In Australia, in June 2005, 46% of children aged 0–12 years received some type of childcare (Australian Bureau of Statistics 2005).

Formal childcare includes preschool, outside hours school care, long daycare, family daycare, occasional and other formal care (Australian Institute of Health and Welfare 2007a). Formal care was utilised by 33% of children in 2005 (Australian Bureau of Statistics 2005). Data for New Zealand date back to a one-off survey in 1998 (Statistics New Zealand 1998), but show a similar rationale as Australia for early childhood education and childcare placement for preschool and school-age children. Three times as many preschool-age children are placed in formal settings than informal settings.

In formal childcare settings there is an emphasis on the child's growth and development, and programs are developed to address their needs. Preschool services are classified as formal childcare. They offer educational and developmental programs to children prior to attending school and are an important aspect of early childhood development. Formal care provides professionally qualified staff and is based on preparing children for school (Australian Institute of Health and Welfare 2007a, Australian Bureau of Statistics 2005).

Informal care refers to non-regulated care that occurs in the child's home or elsewhere. This care is provided by family members, particularly grandparents who provide care for 20% of children, friends, neighbours, and babysitters and nannies. Many parents use a combination of formal and informal childcare (Australian Bureau of Statistics 2005).

Hayden (2002b) suggests that much research and literature in the area of childcare is focused on illness in childcare, reducing the spread of disease, and the incidence of infections within this environment. In addition, many of the relevant policies and guidelines have an illness, rather than health promoting, focus. While staying healthy in childcare is important, and there are useful strategies to limit the spread of infection (National Health and Medical Research Council 2005), this emphasis seems to have overshadowed the opportunities for developing health promoting environments. For current recommendations on exclusion from school, see Box 8.2.

Box 8.2 Practice highlight: exclusion from school guidelines

Exclusion from school and childcare is recommended for a number of infectious illnesses. Access the relevant websites for the current recommendations:

- In Australia, the National Health and Medical Research Council: www.nhmrc.gov.au/publications/synopses/_files/ch43.htm.
- In New Zealand, infectious diseases exclusion information can be found at: www.healthed.govt.nz/resources/infectiousdiseases.aspx.

The school environment

School plays a major part in a child's life, and the school curriculum and school environment are important settings for health promotion. Health Promoting Schools is a worldwide movement developed by the World Health Organization (2007) to support and promote the health and wellbeing of children and young people in schools. While the Health Promoting Schools models began as early as 1950, it was in the 1990s that schools in Australia and New Zealand became involved in the project. The New Zealand Canterbury District Health Board site is recommended to readers (www.cph.co.nz / About-Us / Health-Promoting-Schools.asp). This provides a good introduction and shows the intersection of Maori health concepts with Health Promotion aims. (See Ch 3 for a description of Maori health.)

A Health Promoting School fosters health and learning and is one that constantly strengthens its capacity as a healthy setting for learning (World Health Organization 2007). The model encourages active partnerships between education and health, and collaborates with family and community at a local level. Thus, Health Promoting Schools are strong in localities where these partnerships are established and maintained. Gary, the community nurse in the scenario, recognises the value of developing education and health partnerships, and takes the opportunity to contribute to the project. Using a Health Promoting Schools framework, Gary speaks to the group about relevant health issues for inclusion in the Expo.

Wainwright et al. (2000) and Whitehead (2006) suggest that the role of nurses in schools has been poorly evaluated and has focused on screening, surveillance and health education. The authors suggest an increasing role for nurses in health promotion and argue the need for interventions to be critically evaluated. Whitehead (2006) suggests that nurses need to engage with the Health Promoting Schools movement to build capacity and further emphasise the health promoting role of nurses. It is a pathway to strengths-focused practice.

Growing up healthy: the theme for the Health Expo

The planning group decides that the theme for the Health Expo will be Growing up Healthy, and have decided to focus on the following areas: physical activity and healthy eating, dealing with teasing and bullying, staying safe—where to get help, and preventing injury. Each of these is considered below.

Physical activity and healthy eating

Good nutrition is an important component of healthy development, and depends on having access to healthy foods (Hayden 2002a). This begins in infancy with promotion of breastfeeding, introduction of appropriate foods after 6 months and, later, assisting children to make healthy food choices by having these available to them.

Baur (2004) discusses the role of school canteens in promoting healthy food choices, as well as the school curriculum for promoting healthy eating and activity. This role is becoming increasingly recognised with specific programs being developed to assist school canteens to provide such choices. For example, the New South Wales Healthy School Canteen Strategy highlights a change in nutrition guidelines for school canteens to a government-endorsed approach where the government provides incentives and funding to change to a healthy school canteen policy. They encourage links between school canteens and the community, and aim to model healthy eating to children and families (Bell & Swinburn 2005).

In New Zealand, the Fruit in Schools project aims to increase the consumption of fruit by children (Ministry of Health New Zealand n.d.). The project has two aims. The first is to encourage and support schools in taking a Health Promoting Schools, or whole school community, approach to health (and includes strategies for increasing physical activity, promoting healthy eating, smoke free and sun protection). The second aim is to provide children in high-need groups with a piece of fruit a day. Such an approach provides practical support for children and assists in establishing an interest in healthy eating within the school environment. Further, the program demonstrates the links between health promotion and illness prevention, as a central motivation of the program is cancer prevention.

Pagnini et al. (2006) discuss the importance of promoting healthy eating and increased activity in long daycare centres and preschools. They discuss the opportunity to do this through the provision of food and incorporating messages about healthy eating and physical play into the curriculum. The report viewed these as core missions and highlighted the need to work in close partnerships with parents. This included support, and changing cultural and environmental factors, that influence healthy eating and physical activity. It identified the need for more child-friendly games, activities and books, as well as songs, posters, training for staff and access to health professionals to speak with staff and parents on these issues.

Bailey (2006) suggests that physical education and sport in schools has a number of benefits, and can be understood in terms of child development in the domains of physical, social, affective, lifestyle and cognitive development. Additionally, there are opportunities for children to engage in physical activity in less formal ways. Beighle et al. (2006), for example, studied children's physical activity during recess and found that children engaged in physical activity for the majority of the recess period, indicating opportunities to encourage activity within the school environment. However, gender differences in physical activity are evident, even in primary-school-aged children.

A Western Australian government survey of child and adolescent physical activity and nutrition in 2003 (Department of the Premier and Cabinet WA 2005) showed that primary school girls undertook significantly less physical activity than boys during break periods at school. Both primary-school-aged girls and boys undertook a range of physical activities during a week, both in and around home and at school. The materials provided by the Western Australian Premier's Physical Activity Taskforce demonstrate the multilayered messaging associated with promoting healthy behaviours. Information is provided for teachers, parents, children and parent associations.

School is integral to the lives of children and has a marked influence on their development and learning. Health promotion in schools, therefore, has a wide influence in that it can strengthen families and communities as they work to enhance the health of children.

Teasing and bullying

Bullying is a serious threat to healthy child development and it is purposeful in attempting to injure or inflict discomfort on another (Crothers & Levinson 2004). Often bullying is a means of establishing dominance or maintaining status (Smokowski & Kopasz 2005). It is common in schools and tends to occur repeatedly. It includes name calling, physical assault, threatening, stealing, vandalising, slandering, taunting and excluding (Smokowski & Kopasz 2005 p. 101). Bullying crosses technology boundaries, being communicated via messages on telephones, SMS text and emails, and in chat rooms (Rivers, in Smith 2004). Long-term effects can be devastating, as it creates humiliation and fear for the victim and has detrimental effects on self-image and self-perception.

In both New Zealand and Australia, schools are responsible for ensuring that policies exist and are enforced to minimise bullying, as they provide safe physical and emotional environments for children (Kazmierow 2004).

Health promoting strategies will focus on building skills and strengths in children, appropriate to their age. Holistic system-based approaches are promoted to create positive school environments. However, the motivations for bullying are numerous and can affect strategies that may be helpful. For example, in earlier childhood, behaviour that is labelled bullying is most likely physical. Greater social development usually sees this sort of assertion of self over others diminish, but emotional bullying may increase. Promoting good self-esteem and assertion in children may diminish emotional bullying (Rigby 2003).

Staying safe—where to get help

While early childhood is a time of activity, learning and fun, children are often faced with difficult circumstances. Many face difficult relationships with family or friends. Bullying and child abuse have been identified as the major reason for younger children contacting help lines (Boystown 2005). If children are not in nurturing or supportive family environments, or if those environments are in crisis, young children rarely have intrinsic or external resources to cope effectively (Boystown 2005). Telephone counselling lines are a last resort for children. Nurses' advocacy role and legal obligations are discussed in detail in Chapter 4.

Being a victim of, or witnessing, violence is a significant reason for children to seek help. Often they experience physical, emotional or sexual abuse. Research into domestic violence has identified preschoolers as blaming themselves for the violence, having sleep disturbances, anxiety and social isolation. Primary-school-aged children also experience difficulties with school, both attending and doing the work, problems concentrating, fighting with peers, rebelling against authority, aggression, depression, and girls particularly being withdrawn and anxious (Gevers 1999 p. 17).

Domestic violence is multidimensional and influenced not only by the violence, but also by separation from a parent, frequent moves, age, sex and the child's personality. It puts these children at risk, in both the short and the long term (Gevers 1999 p. 17). Some children learn to use violence as a way of solving problems. All domestic violence is traumatic and has chronic long-term impacts on the child psychologically, whether as a victim or as a witness to it (Gevers 1999, National Association for Prevention of Child Abuse and Neglect n.d.). Violence is a complex issue, but an important one for health promotion action in schools and communities.

Talking about bodies, sexuality and self-protection is important in the early years. Box 8.3 describes a recently developed resource to assist parents and teachers.

Box 8.3 Critical questions and reflections: talking about bodies

In April 2007, Family Planning Queensland (FPQ) published a children's book titled *Everyone's got a bottom*. The storybook for children aged 3–8 years is about Ben and his brother and sister learning and talking about bodies. It is designed as a tool for parents and carers to begin to talk about bodies and self-protection. The book is part of FPQ's long-term plan to provide evidence-based child protection education.

The publication met mixed reactions with some media coverage suggesting that the book was too detailed.

Access the storybook: T Rowley and J Edwards 2007 *Everyone's got a bottom*. Family Planning Queensland.

1. How might you introduce the book to children and parents?
2. Reflect on the language and content of the book. Consider how your personal values and judgments influence your appraisal of the tool.

Preventing injury

The inquisitive, exploratory nature of young children means that injuries and accidents are common. Many are preventable; some are inevitable. The 0–14-year age group has been identified as the group most likely to sustain an injury, with 25% being reported in this group (Australian Bureau of Statistics 2006a). The most common were cuts at 28%, falls below one metre 55%, falls more than one metre 51%, attacks by other people 51%, and 37% from bites or stings. Of these injuries, 54% occurred during leisure time, sports activities comprised 15%, and 12% occurred while at school (Australian Bureau of Statistics 2006a). The risk of injuries at home is more common in younger children, and boys have been found to be at higher risk of injury than girls, and this proportion increases with age (Kendrick et al. 2007).

Unintentional poisoning, childhood falls, pedestrian injuries, burns and passenger injuries are all cited as common injuries in the New Zealand data (Safekids New Zealand n.d.). In a study of fractures in New Zealand elementary school settings, Rubie-Davies and Townsend (2007) found that across 76 schools (over 25,000 students) in a 1-year period, 118 students sustained a total of 131 fractures. Compared to international data, this rate is low, but, interestingly, fewer fractures were involved in playground equipment than expected. The researchers suggest that injury may be influenced more by the way students interact than the safety of equipment.

The Health Expo suggested in the scenario is a way to provide a school with the opportunity to share information and showcase strategies in a number of child health areas. Promoting healthy development in early childhood is a key to prevention and to promoting resilience, strength and wellbeing in young children. It is a means of building on the protective factors they have and protecting them from intrinsic and extrinsic risks and vulnerabilities (see Table 1.1 in Ch 1). However, these years are often marked by episodes of acute illness. The second part of the chapter discusses the contexts of care for childhood acute illness episodes.

Setting the scene: an acute illness episode

Ethan is 3 years old. His parents Meena and Napo also have a daughter, Ruby, who is 5 years old and has just started school. Meena works 2 days a week, while Napo works fulltime. When Meena is at work, Ethan attends a local childcare centre. Ethan has been a well and happy baby. Meena breastfed him for 12 months. He has had few illnesses, although he has had mild eczema since he was weaned. Over the past week, both Ethan and Ruby have had a respiratory infection.

Meena is disturbed by Ethan's fitful crying during his afternoon nap. Ethan is sitting up in bed, and struggling for breath. He is very pale, and trying to cry, but is having trouble getting air in and out. Meena notices that the spaces between his ribs become obvious with each breath and realises that she needs information and help. She bundles the children into the car and drives to her local general practice surgery, which is only 10 minutes away. There the practice nurse assesses Ethan, noting his pallor, respiratory rate and character, and pulse rate.

The practice nurse then consults with the general practitioner who, in turn, assesses the child. They agree that he is best treated in hospital, and organise his transfer to the emergency department and ambulance transport. He spends 2 hours in the emergency department of the children's hospital being monitored and treated. He is discharged home with medication, a regime for its administration, and information for Meena concerning his care and condition.

The next day she takes him back to the general practitioner for a follow-up consultation and assessment. Ethan has had a first asthma episode and will need a specialist referral.

Describing acute childhood illness

An acute illness in children may be described as one that is of rapid onset, has severe symptoms and is of brief duration (Neill 2005). In the main, children will be cared for at home by their family. It is only when a child is unstable, becomes very ill, or requires surgical intervention, that hospital admission is needed.

Children in Australia and New Zealand suffer from a range of acute illnesses, but patterns of childhood illness have changed over time. Looking back to the 1950s, for example, there is a picture of infectious diseases dominating childhood illness such as poliomyelitis, measles, chicken pox, mumps and rubella (among others).

Such illnesses, while expected events of a child's life, had little or no treatment, and, at times, had ongoing and even catastrophic complications, ranging from deafness, infertility and physical disability, to paralysis, brain damage and death. With the development of effective preventive medicine via vaccination, the risk of these diseases has been negated or minimised in most developed countries.

Today, by comparison, children in countries such as Australia and New Zealand are most likely to experience acute illness from a very different range of sources, such as unintentional injury, issues arising from the perinatal period (e.g. complications of prematurity), or those related to environmental effects ranging from gastrointestinal infections to obesity and respiratory conditions (including asthma). In some sections of the childhood populations of both countries, ear infections remain a significant acute illness. This includes Aboriginal and Torres Strait Islander and Maori children who tend to have poorer health and a higher incidence of specific illnesses and injuries than other groups (Australian Institute of Health and Welfare 2007b, New Zealand Health Information Service 2007). In Chapter 3, a full discussion of Aboriginal and Torres Strait Islander peoples and Maori health is provided.

A further factor to consider is that the type and incidence of acute illnesses differs according to age. Respiratory illnesses present the most common cause for hospital admissions for infants in both New Zealand and Australia. Respiratory illnesses continue as a significant cause of hospitalisation in older children (Australian Institute of Health and Welfare 2007b, New Zealand Health Information Service 2007). Infants and toddlers have a greater incidence of non-specific febrile illnesses, gastrointestinal illnesses and some respiratory viral illnesses than other age groups.

Young children under 5 are the age group most likely to have health consequences from unintentional injury (Kidsafe WA n.d., Safekids New Zealand n.d.). Unintentional injury is a significant source of acute illness and is the most common cause of childhood hospitalisation and death in New Zealand in children aged 0–14 (Safekids New Zealand n.d.). In Australia, only respiratory illnesses are a greater cause of hospitalisation for children than injury. The sources of injury include motor vehicle and cycle-related accidents, falls, fire injury, cuts and abrasions, and poisons. Again the distribution or these injuries varies with age group.

Contexts of care for children with acute illness

Looking at the scenario, it is clear that Ethan's illness is treated and cared for in more than one context or setting. In fact, three are evident in the story: the home, general practice and hospital. Each of these settings is examined below, not only in the context of the clinical scenario, but also more broadly, as each relates to caring for children with acute illness.

Care for a child at home

Often when a child becomes ill, they are cared for at home with little or no medical intervention. In this setting, care is most often by family, usually a parent. (For our purposes, 'parent' is defined as the person who is the primary caregiver to a child.)

This can present specific issues for families, beyond those related to assessment and treatment of their sick child. Parents like Ethan's are likely to have to consider reorganising their work outside the home and other family activities. A parent may need to stay home from work. Alternatively, a friend, relative or paid carer may need to be organised to come to the home. Childcare or school will need to be notified of the child's absence.

In Australia, 57% of mothers work (Australian Bureau of Statistics 2006b), and, in New Zealand, 78% of partnered women with dependent children and 58% of sole mothers are employed outside the home (Statistics New Zealand 2005). Further, in New Zealand, Maori women have the highest rates of participation in unpaid work outside the household and looking after children in the home (Statistics New Zealand 2005). The rates of workforce participation by women are significantly lower for families with infants and toddlers.

It is interesting to note that, in Sweden, all parents have the ability to take 60 days per year on 80% of their salary to care for sick children (Shields 2000). Such generous allowances are not available in Australia or New Zealand and a child's illness, whether treated at home or in hospital, is a family stressor. How parents appraise the situation and what and how they use available resources may determine how well the family copes with the situation.

If a child is cared for at home, parents, other family and carers assess, monitor and treat the child, and so good knowledge of the child's presentation and needs will be important. It is important that a child rests, drinks plenty of fluid, and has a subsequent normal urine output. The child may not be hungry, but nutrition can be given through light drinks. A parent will know by touch if a child has a high temperature. Current research advocates that a fever be allowed to run its course (Russell et al. 2003), and that disease processes can be prolonged if a fever is dampened by antipyretic medication (Lagerløv et al. 2006). However, children often feel better after a dose of paracetamol or a similar drug (approved for use with children) to relieve the malaise that accompanies a high temperature, so parents may have to choose which course of action to take. It is important for anyone who is sick to rest, and children will naturally want to sleep if they feel ill.

Recall in the scenario that Meena's initial assessment of her sick child led her to seek medical help. Parents' decisions about when to seek assistance for their child's illness are influenced by a range of circumstances. With minor illness, the wait-and-see approach is often used (Allen et al. 2002). If the child remains ill, they may consult a range of health services (Neill 2005). In a recent survey of Australian parents, telephone advice was the most popular source of input in both less acute and emergency situations (Keatinge 2006). The general practitioner was the next most commonly used source of advice, with the child health clinic the least often used.

In a study conducted in Western Australia, a correlation was found to exist between mothers' use of both general practitioner and hospital services and that of their children, suggesting an intergenerational correlation (Ward et al. 2006). This infers that one's parents may influence the actions one takes as a parent. Parents may also take their sick child to a hospital emergency department if they are dissatisfied with the diagnosis or service given by a general practitioner (Ryan et al. 2005). Along with telephone advice, emergency department advice is also used during out-of-office hours.

Given the responsibilities borne by parents in assessing and treating a sick or injured child, the significance of universal preventive health services and information initiatives in contributing to support for their efforts cannot be overstressed. Community-based information about childhood illness and injury, treatment options and contacts, and sources of information and advice that are accessible and appropriate, are critical resources.

Community care

Although community services for children vary, recent moves in short-stay hospitalisation have seen the development of 'hospital-in-the-home' or 'hospital-at-home' schemes. These were first suggested in the 1970s. Shepperd and Ilife (2005) define hospital at home as:

> '. . . a service that provides active treatment by health care professionals, in the patient's home, of a condition that otherwise would require acute hospital in-patient care, always for a limited period'.

Early discharge is the most widely researched area of hospital-at-home initiatives. Research has shown that these schemes bring increased satisfaction with care, and no known adverse effects (Cooper et al. 2006). Such schemes in the United Kingdom have been shown to be effective and cost neutral to the National Health Service (Bagust et al. 2002), and this has been confirmed in an Australian study of adult hospital-at-home services (MacIntyre et al. 2002). However, the economic benefits of such programs over in-hospital care are contended (Shepperd & Ilife 2005).

Specially prepared paediatric nurses visit children and their families in their homes to:

1. assist with the child's illness, and
2. increase the understanding and confidence of parents who are caring for their child (Neill 2005).

The child may have been sent home from hospital with intravenous therapy *in situ*, they may have a variety of acute illnesses, and the nursing team is available 24 hours per day, 7 days a week. As well as routine visits, parents can, in the first instance, call the nurses by telephone, and on triage the nurse gives advice, or refers the child to the general practitioner or arranges for a visit by a nurse. In Chapter 12, the needs of a child, Tihema, and her family, as she goes home from hospital but with ongoing dependence on medical technology and healthcare, are discussed. This presents an example of hospital-at-home in the context of ongoing, or chronic, illness and the transfer of care responsibilities to family carers with professional support.

Another community approach to caring for children with an acute illness is ambulatory care. Ambulatory care is an innovation that has developed as the cost of hospital inpatient services has grown. In an attempt to cut length of stay, and prevent unnecessary admission, ambulatory care units have been set up in many hospitals. A child (or adult) arrives for care in the hospital, but is not fully admitted; rather, they are kept in an 'admissions ward', sometimes for up to 12 hours, for observation or minor treatment, and then sent home in the care of the well-prepared parent(s). Ambulatory care is said to increase parental satisfaction, and save costs (Woolfenden et al. 2005). In addition to ambulatory care as described, there is ongoing development in the area of telemedicine to provide innovate care for children and families. Box 8.4 describes the use of technology in healthcare for children.

Box 8.4 Practice highlight: paediatric telemedicine

Modern technology is providing new ways of delivering care to children and families. Telephone triage, where parents can ring and discuss a child's condition with a nurse who then refers them to a doctor, advises on care at home, or advises on admission to hospital, has been in place in the Nordic countries as a first point of entry to the health service for many years (Shields 2000), and has been successfully implemented in Australia (Hanson et al. 2004) and in New Zealand (St George & Cullen 2001).

Based at the Royal Children's Hospital in Brisbane is the University of Queensland's telemedicine service (www.uq.edu.au/coh/). This is being successfully used to provide healthcare and diagnostic services across the state. It has been used for palliative care for children with cancer and other illnesses (Pensink et al. 2004), the delivery of burns care to rural and remote areas (Smith et al. 2004), and for preadmission screening of children undergoing ear, nose and throat surgery (Smith et al. 2004). Parents who could attend a videoconference rather than an outpatient clinic appointment found that the videoconferencing reduced their costs, as they did not have to pay for parking, petrol and meals (Smith et al. 2004).

Information about New Zealand telemedicine programs can also be accessed by going to www.starship.org.nz/index.php/pi_pageid/1464.

When an admission to hospital is needed

Ethan was treated in the emergency department of a hospital. If he had been admitted as an inpatient, he would have entered an unfamiliar and unusual environment. He and his family would have required particular attention to help them familiarise themselves with the environment and cope with the stress of admission. His parents would need assistance to understand their role in his care in an environment so different from home.

Ideally, children are able to visit a hospital for a preadmission visit to enable them to become familiar with the sights and sounds of a hospital (Rollins 1999). Of course, this is impossible if children are admitted as an emergency, but, for more routine admissions, such schemes have been found to be invaluable. However, health services across the world are restricting such services, as they are costly to run. A flexible approach to such programs is needed that integrates supportive technologies, reduces costs, increases access from home for children to such programs, and provides effective and cost-efficient ways to prepare children for a hospital admission (Mitchell et al. 2004).

While there has been a decline in preadmission programs for children, other methods of introducing children to hospital have been developing. For example, the 'teddy bear hospital' is gaining favour (www.teddybearhospital.com.au/). The staff visit schools and children bring their teddy bears to school on that day. The children present their sick teddy bears to the staff, who act as nurses and doctors to discuss with the children the teddy bears' problems, and in this way break down barriers and ameliorate children's fears of hospitals and health services (Toker et al. 2002).

The internet provides a new access point to information for children and their parents and families, not only about going to hospital but, more generally, to gain information and assistance with their healthcare needs. Internet-based resources have been developed by a number of the larger public children's hospitals in New Zealand and Australia, and it is recommended that the reader look up the resources available for their local major facilities (see Box 8.5).

Box 8.5 Critical questions and reflections: preparing for hospital

Look at the websites for children's hospitals in New Zealand and Australia, perhaps starting with facilities in your state or Health Board District. Two excellent examples are:

1. the Starship Hospital in Auckland (www.starship.org.nz/index.php/ps_pagename/homepage), which provides inpatient and outpatient services for children, as well as coordinating community child health and home paediatric services, and
2. the Melbourne Royal Children's Hospital (www.rch.org.au/rch/index.cfm?doc_id=1495), which provides parents and families with information about going to hospital, childhood illness and support. Children can access information and can see activities available for and undertaken by children at the hospital.

Also keep in mind the information about young children's development that you read earlier in this chapter and look up information about age-appropriate communication strategies in Chapter 5.

After spending time looking, reading and reflecting, try to devise a program or resource package that might assist a family such as Ethan's if he were admitted as an inpatient. While you might be thinking about content, also think about priorities as they might be viewed from a child's point of view, and from a family's point of view. Think about the possible presentation formats you could use, weighing up their advantages and limitations to meet your goals.

Balancing children's and parents' needs

At the hospital bedside, children and parents have needs. Understanding these needs provides a lens through which nurses can approach care for the child. Children's needs for nurturing, continuity and security are universal. Other needs are more age specific. For example, one study of hospitalised boys' needs (Runeson et al. 2002) presented four categories of need: the need for control, the need to have parents nearby, the need for what is familiar, and the need for integrity. Coyne (2006) points out that children need to be informed in a way that is appropriate to their age. Coyne found that providing information about illness and treatments helped primary and older age children to feel a greater sense of control and involvement. Yet even a young child, such as Ethan, needs to have information about his experience and situation.

Parents' needs have also been examined. One study (Kristjánsdóttir 1995) identified six categories of parent needs:

1. to be able to trust doctors and nurses
2. information

3. the presence of other family members
4. to feel they are trusted
5. support and guidance, and
6. physical needs.

These themes are consistent across cultures (Shields et al. 2004) and are useful for developing a communication framework when working with parents. To examine these concepts further, read the research highlight in Box 8.6 and attempt the reader activity.

Box 8.6 Research highlight: parental participation

A study by O'Haire and Blackford (2005) investigated the experiences of nurses negotiating parental participation in the care of their hospitalised child. A grounded theory approach was used. Data were collected through individual interviews, document analysis and focus group. The main phenomenon identified was that of moral agency. Causal to this were the best interests of the child and disputes about care and the nurses' expectations. Specific categories identified through analysis were:

- moral agency (the central phenomenon)
- the child's best interests
- disputes about care
- nurses' expectations of parents
- moral distress, and
- coping mechanisms and strategies.

The concept of moral agency refers to the desire among participants to deliver the best care possible. However, from the analysis, a number of situations threatened this sense of moral agency. For example, when parents and nurses disagreed about care and when nurses' expectations of parents were not met, there was potential for conflict and indeed the provision of suboptimal care.

Reader activity

Consider how the findings of the research could influence practice. Apply the principles of practice development with the goal of changing practice and culture to improve parental participation in care.

Family-centred care in hospitals

The approach to care adopted for a child like Ethan and his family, or any child admitted to hospital as either an urgent and unexpected or an expected event embeds some important principles. These are needed in order to facilitate the child's recovery from illness and support the wellbeing of the child and family. Family-centred care (FCC) is one approach or model that has been influential in the care of children in hospital.

FCC, as an approach to caring for children in hospital, was developed over a number of years and grounded in the original work of John Bowlby in the 1950s, when the essential role of parenting and the family in a child's care and health were recognised along with the negative emotional effects of hospitalisation for children, infants and young children in particular. Over a number of years, consumer organisations, such as the Association for the Welfare of Child Health (n.d.) (formerly the Association for the Welfare of Children in Hospital), have influenced policy and practice, increasing the involvement of parents and family in caring for their hospitalised children.

In short, the practice of excluding parents and family from the hospital bedside except for very restricted periods has been replaced by inclusive practice, whereby parents and family are included and essential to decision making. In theory, at least, nursing care complements parent care (Franck & Callery 2004).

Research into family-centred practice and the associated concepts of parental participation, parental involvement in care, partnership with parents and care by parents has shown the complexity of turning the theory and ideals of family-centred practice into reality (Darbyshire 1994, Alsop-Shields 2002). Just how parents and nurses share the care and responsibility for a hospitalised child remains contentious (Franck & Callery 2004, Paliadelis et al. 2005). One qualitative study suggested that nurses have a positive orientation to FCC. However, they struggle with understandings about their own professional and expert role and how this fits with the role of parents (Palliadelis et al. 2005). In addition, this study identified organisational features that nurses perceived negatively affected their ability to implement FCC. Elements common to many nursing contexts were identified, including workload, staff skill mix and staffing levels.

The tensions surrounding both the theory and practice of FCC have been explored by Franck and Callery (2004). They identified a number of problematic aspects of the approach, including the interpretation of concepts, implementation, and differences between lay and professional knowledge. Further, they raise the important issue of the interests of the child and how these need to be kept central. The point is made (p. 269) that the:

> '. . . difference between "child-centred" and "family-centred" care is one of emphasis: neither term can exclude the other, because child-centred care must take account of the social environment in which children live and FCC must be primarily concerned with the health of children'.

Further, they argue the need for research to be theoretically sound and propose a conceptual framework for examining FCC in different clinical settings (p. 271). In the case of Ethan's care for asthma, the framework might be applied in the following way:

1. *Child/family empowerment*. The family would have good knowledge of the symptoms and the therapies and develop confidence in managing Ethan's asthma. At age 3, Ethan would be able to communicate if he feels unwell and accept treatments as something to make him better or breathe easier.
2. *Support of family healthcare for child*. The family attends follow-up with general practice and specialists and shows an acceptance and adjustment to Ethan's asthma.
3. *Child/family-friendly health services/individualised care*. It will be clear that an educational process is undertaken with the family, perhaps with a liaison nurse from the hospital and/or general practice nurse.

4. *Participation in care.* Ethan's family monitors his progress and symptoms and takes appropriate treatment actions when needed. They might keep a journal to assist them.
5. *Shared healthcare decision making.* Ethan's parents participate in consultations with all health professionals. Their knowledge and goals for Ethan are sought out by professionals and included in planning, and they are an integral part of communication among hospital and general practice professionals.

This example demonstrates that approaches to caring for young children with an acute illness episode are multidimensional. Being child and family centred is a complex practice dependent not only on bedside communication but also on the overarching care for the child's condition, before, during and after a hospital visit.

Conclusion

Early childhood is a time of growth, learning and play in which children demonstrate rapidly developing psychosocial, emotional, physical and cognitive competence. Promoting health and wellbeing for children and their families is an important health service focus that can influence longer term health and wellbeing, and, more broadly, the strength of communities. Health promoting services can be undertaken across a range of settings. These include schools, community centres and childcare centres, through internet resources for children and families, and through strategic programs implemented with intersectoral collaboration.

For nurses working with young children, the ability to think outside the box, challenge silo culture and harness children's curiosity and appetite for exploring and learning are key challenges for practice in the twenty-first century. Whether nurses are working with well children and their families or with children experiencing an acute illness episode, strengthening the child and family through collaborative approaches to practice, in ways that maintain the balance of both child and family centredness, are current underpinnings and the directions for the future.

Practice tips

- Childcare and school environments are natural settings for health promotion.
- Early childhood is a time when patterns of healthy eating and activity can be modelled.
- Collaborate with parents and communities to develop healthy school environments.
- Most care for acutely ill children is provided by the family.
- Consider the needs of both the child and family when hospitalisation is needed.
- Reflect critically on nurses' professional role and how this might be used to complement parents' care of their child.
- Healthcare for young children needs to balance 'child' centredness with 'family' centredness at all levels, from policy to direct caregiving, no matter what its context—clinic, telephone, internet or hospital.

Useful resources

KIA KAHA No bully: www.police.govt.nz/service/yes/nobully/kia_kaha/.
Kidsafe: www.kidsafevic.com.au.
Kids Help Line: www.kidshelp.com.au.
Melbourne Royal Children's Hospital: www.rch.org.au/rch/index.cfm?doc_id=1495.
National Association for the Prevention of Child Abuse and Neglect (NAPCAN): http://napcan.org.au.
National Child Protection Clearinghouse publications: www.aifs.gov.au/nch.
National Health and Medical Research Council: www.nhmrc.gov.au/publications.
No Bully: www.nobully.org.nz/advicep.htm.
Safekids New Zealand: www.safekids.org.nz/index.php/ps.
Starship Children's Hospital Auckland: www.starship.org.nz.

References

Allen J, Dyas J, Jones M 2002 Minor illnesses in children: parents' views and use of health services. *Journal of Community Nursing* 7:462–8.

Alsop-Shields L 2002 The parent–staff interaction model of pediatric care. *Journal of Pediatric Nursing* 17(6):442–9.

Association for the Welfare of Child Health (AWCH) n.d. Available at www.awch.org.au/about.html.

Australian Bureau of Statistics (ABS) 2005 *Child care Australia June 2005* (reissue). ABS, Canberra. Available at www.abs.gov.au/AUSSTATS/abs@.nsf/ProductsbyReleaseDate/03D307053D1C.

Australian Bureau of Statistics (ABS) 2006a *Injury in Australia: a snapshot 2004–2005*. Available at www.abs.gov.au/Ausstats/abs@.nsf/39433889d406eeb9ca2570610019e9a5/7b18.

Australian Bureau of Statistics (ABS) 2006b *Trends in women's employment: the proportion of women who were employed increased in every age group between 1979 and 2004*. Cat. No. 4102.0. Available at www.abs.gov.au/ausstats/abs@.nsf/7d12b0f6763c78caca257061001cc588/858badad39afb98dca2571b000153d73!OpenDocument. Accessed 3 February 2007.

Australian Institute of Health and Welfare (AIHW) 2007a *Final report on the development of the children's services national minimum data set*. Cat. No. CFS 6. AIHW, Canberra.

Australian Institute of Health and Welfare (AIHW) 2007b *National hospital morbidity database separation, patient day and average length of stay statistics by principal diagnosis in ICD-10-AM, Australia, 1998–99 to 2004–05*. Available at www.aihw.gov.au/cognos/cgi-bin/ppdscgi?DC=Q&E=/ahs/principaldiagnosis9899-0405. Accessed 7 January 2007.

Bagust A, Haycox A, Sartain S 2002 Economic evaluation of an acute paediatric hospital at home clinical trial. *Archives of Disease in Childhood* 87:489–92.

Bailey R 2006 Physical education and sport in schools: a review of benefits and outcomes. *Journal of School Health* 76(8):397–401.

Baur L 2004 The epidemic of childhood obesity: what roles do schools play in primary prevention? *Nutrition and Dietetics* 61(3):134–5.

Beighle A, Morgan C, Le Masurier G, Pangrazi R 2006 Children's physical activity during recess and outside of school. *Journal of School Health* 76(10):516–20.

Bell A, Swinburn B 2005 School canteens: using ripples to create a wave of healthy eating. *Medical Journal of Australia* 183(1):5–6.

Boystown 2005 *Kids Help Line 2005 overview: what is concerning children and young people in Australia?* Available at www.kidshelp.com.au.

Cooper C, Wheeler DM, Woolfenden SR et al. 2006 Specialist home-based nursing services for children with acute and chronic illnesses. Cochrane Database of Systematic Reviews. Issue 4, Art. No. CD004383.

Coyne I 2006 Consultation with children in hospital: children, parents' and nurses' perspectives. *Journal of Clinical Nursing* 15:61–71.

Crothers L, Levinson E 2004 Assessment of bullying: a review of methods and instruments. *Journal of Counseling and Development* 82:496–503.

Darbyshire P 1994 *Living with a sick child in hospital, the experiences of parents and nurses*. Chapman & Hall, London.

Department of the Premier and Cabinet WA 2005 *Children and adolescent physical activity and nutrition survey 2003*. Available at www.patf.dpc.wa.gov.au/index.cfm?event=resources#CAPANSfs.

Franck LS, Callery P 2004 Re-thinking family centred care across the continuum of children's health care. *Child: Care, Health and Development* 30(3):265–77.

Gevers L 1999 *Kids and DV. Practice standards for working with children and young people who have lived with domestic violence*. Families, Youth and Community Care, Queensland.

Hanson RM, Exley BJ, Ngo P et al. 2004 Paediatric telephone triage and advice: the demand continues. *Medical Journal of Australia* 180:333–5.

Hayden J 2002a Nutrition and child development: global perspectives. *Child Care Information Exchange* 5(02):38–41.

Hayden J 2002b Revisiting the early childhood-health dyad: health promotion in early childhood settings—implications for policy and practice. *Delta* 54(1/2):57–71.

Kazmierow M 2004 *Bullying in schools and the law*. Available at http://nzplc.massey.ac.nz/default.asp?page=docs/bullymain.htm. Accessed 1 April 2007.

Keatinge D 2006 Parents' preferred child health information sources: implications for nursing practice. *Australian Journal of Advanced Nursing* 23:13–18.

Kendrick D, Coupland C, Mulvaney C et al. 2007 *Home safety education and provision of safety equipment for injury prevention*. Cochrane Database of Systematic Reviews. Issue 1, Art. No. CD005014. DOI:10.1002/14651858.CD005014.pub2.

Kidsafe WA n.d. Child Accident Prevention Foundation of Australia website. Available at www.kidsafewa.com.au/.

Kristjánsdóttir G 1995 Perceived importance of needs expressed by parents of hospitalized two- to six-year olds. *Scandinavian Journal of Caring Sciences* 9:95–103.

Lagerløv P, Loeb M, Slettevoll J et al. 2006 Severity of illness and the use of paracetamol in febrile preschool children; a case simulation study of parents' assessments. *Family Practice* 23:618–23.

MacIntyre CR, Ruth D, Ansari Z 2002 Hospital in the home is cost saving for appropriately selected patients: a comparison with in-hospital care. *International Journal for Quality in Health Care* 14:285–93.

Ministry of Health New Zealand (MOH NZ) n.d. *Fruit in schools*. Available at www.moh.govt.nz/fruitinschools.

Mitchell M, Johnston L, Keppell M 2004 Preparing children and their families for hospitalisation: a review of the literature. *Neonatal, Paediatric and Child Health Nursing* 7:5–15.

National Association for Prevention of Child Abuse and Neglect (NAPCAN) n.d. Available at www.napcan.org.au / about.htm.

National Health and Medical Research Council (NHMRC) 2005 *Staying healthy in child care. Preventing infectious diseases in child care*, 4th edn. NHMRC, Canberra. Available at www.nhmrc.gov.au / publications / synopses / _files / ch43.pdf.

Neill S 2005 Caring for the acutely ill child at home. In A Sidey & D Widdas, *Textbook of community children's nursing*. Elsevier, Edinburgh, pp. 237–48.

New Zealand Health Information Service 2007 *Table 1: Discharges from publicly funded hospitals—chapters, subgroups and individual 3 digit ICD-10 codes by sex and age 2002–3*. Available at www.nzhis.govt.nz / stats / index.html. Accessed 7 January 2007.

Oates K, Currow K, Hu W 2001 *Child health. A practical manual for general practice*. MacLennan & Petty, Sydney.

O'Haire S, Blackford J 2005 Nurses' moral agency in negotiating parental participation in care. *International Journal of Nursing Practice* 11:250–6.

Pagnini D, Wilkenfeld R, King L et al. 2006 *The weight of opinion: the early childhood sector's perceptions about childhood overweight and obesity*. NSW Centre for Overweight and Obesity, Sydney.

Paliadelis P, Cruickshank M, Wainohu D et al. 2005 Implementing family-centred care: an exploration of the beliefs and practices of paediatric nurses. *Australian Journal of Advanced Nursing* 23(1):31–6.

Pensink M, Arnfield N, Russell TG et al. 2004 Paediatric palliative home care with internet-based video phones: lesson learnt. *Journal of Telemedicine and Telecare* 10(Suppl 1):10–13.

Rigby K 2003 *Addressing bullying in schools: theory and practice. Trends and issues in crime and criminal justice*. Australian Institute of Criminology. Available at www.aic.gov.au / publications / . Accessed 10 April 2007.

Rollins JR 1999 Family-centered care of the child during illness and hospitalization. In DL Wong, M Hockenberry-Eaton & ML Winkelstein et al. (eds), *Whaley & Wong's nursing care of infants and children*, 6th edn. Mosby, St Louis, pp. 1131–209.

Rowley T, Edwards J 2007 *Everyone's got a bottom*. Family Planning Queensland.

Rubie-Davies CM, Townsend MA 2007 Fractures in New Zealand elementary school settings. *Journal of School Health* 77(1):36–40.

Runeson I, Hallström I, Elander G, Hermeren G 2002 Children's needs during hospitalization: an observational study of hospitalized boys. *International Journal of Nursing Practice* 8:158–66.

Russell FM, Shann F, Curtis N, Mulholland K 2003 Evidence on the use of paracetamol in febrile children. *Bulletin of the World Health Organization* 81:367–72.

Ryan M, Spicer M, Hyett C, Barnett P 2005 Non-urgent presentations to a paediatric emergency department: parental behaviours, expectations and outcomes emergency. *Medicine Australasia* 17:457–62.

Safekids New Zealand n.d *Injury data*. Available at www.safekids.org.nz / index.php / ps_pagename / injurydata.

Shepperd S, Iliffe S 2005 *Hospital at home versus in-patient hospital care*. Cochrane Database of Systematic Reviews. Issue 3, Art. No. CD000356. DOI: 10.1002 / 14651858.CD000356.pub2.

Sheridan MD 1994 *From birth to five years. Children's developmental progress*. ACER, Melbourne.

Shields L 2000 *The delivery of family-centred care in hospitals in Iceland, Sweden and England: a report for the Winston Churchill Memorial Trust 2001*. Available at www.churchilltrust.com.au/res/File/Fellow_Reports/Shields%20Linda%202000.pdf. Accessed 16 February 2007.

Shields L, Hunter J, Hall J 2004 Parents' and staff's perceptions of parental needs during a child's admission to hospital: an English perspective. *Journal of Child Health Care* 8:9–33.

Smith AC, Youngberry K, Kimble R, Wootton R 2004 A review of three years experience using email and videoconferencing for the delivery of post-acute burns care to children in Queensland. *Burns* 30:248–52.

Smith P 2004 Bullying: recent developments. *Child and Adolescent Mental Health* 9(3):98–103.

Smokowski P, Kopasz K 2005 Bullying in school: an overview of types, effects, family characteristics, and intervention strategies. *National Association of Social Workers* 27(2):101–10.

Statistics New Zealand 1998 *Childcare, families and work: the New Zealand childcare survey*. Joint project of the Department of Labour and the National Advisory Council on the Employment of Women (NACEW). Available at www.nacew.govt.nz/publications/nz-childcare-survey.doc.

Statistics New Zealand 2005 *Focusing on women*. Available at www.stats.govt.nz/NR/rdonlyres/FC1BDDF4-F40F-4B05-B00C-104AC9D38D78/0/FocusingOnWomen2005.pdf.

St George IK, Cullen MJ 2001 The Healthline pilot: call centre triage in New Zealand. *New Zealand Medical Journal* 114:429–30.

Toker A, Urkin J, Boch Y 2002 Role of a medical students' association in improving the curriculum at a faculty of health sciences. *Medical Teacher* 24:634–6.

Wainwright P, Thomas J, Jones M 2000 Health promotion and the role of the school nurse: systematic review. *Journal of Advanced Nursing* 32(5):1083–91.

Ward AM, Klerk N, Pritchard D et al. 2006 Correlations of siblings' and mothers' utilisation of primary and hospital health care: a record linkage study in Western Australia. *Social Science and Medicine* 62:1341–8.

Whitehead D 2006 The health-promoting school: what role for nursing? *Journal of Clinical Nursing* 15:264–71.

Wong D, Perry S, Hockenberry M et al. 2006 *Maternal child nursing care*, 3rd edn. Mosby Elsevier, St Louis.

Woolfenden SP, Dalkeith T, Anderson T 2005 The first eighteen months of a paediatric ambulatory and community service. *Australian Health Review* 29: 429–34.

World Health Organization (WHO) 2007 *What is a Health Promoting School?* Available at www.who.int/school_youth_health/gshi/hps/en/.

Chapter 9

The young person

Lindsay Smith

Learning outcomes

Reading this chapter will help you to:

- » identify three key strategies for providing best nursing care of the young person
- » understand the importance of the bioecological context of the young person
- » review key indicators of health and wellbeing for the young person in Australia and New Zealand
- » discuss a range of protective factors that support health and development for the young person
- » discuss a range of risks that threaten health and development for the young person
- » discuss the broad bioecological determinants that influence health and development for the young person
- » describe how nurses can promote health and support optimal outcomes for the young person in the community
- » identify four important stages that a relationship moves through and some actions that enhance connectedness with young people
- » discuss how nurses can enhance personal, family and community strengths to support optimum health and development for the young person
- » conduct a nursing assessment of family strengths with a young person, and
- » recognise the challenges that you the nurse may experience in caring for the young person.

Introduction

This chapter explores nursing the young person within the context of their family and their community. The focus of this chapter is to understand how nurses promote health and wellbeing for the young person across the bioecological context. The life stage between late childhood and young adulthood (approximately 10–24 years old) is together termed the 'young person' in this chapter. Our understanding of this period of life is changing, especially in relation to adolescence. Many children are moving out of the innocence and dependence of childhood at a younger age. Likewise, it may take longer for adolescents to move fully away from semidependence on their family. Thus, nursing young people is not bound by age and hormonal changes of the person (as much as these bring significant biological factors that need to be considered) as it is bound by fulfilling their personal achievement and autonomy within specific sociocultural contexts.

The young person lives through an exciting period of life that is characterised by transitions. Through these transitions, from one developmental achievement to the next, emerge challenges that the young person needs to address successfully so they emerge as a young adult established for a successful life journey. These transitions are all about potential—potential of what the young person may achieve and become. The bioecological theory of human development (Bronfenbrenner 2001) argues that inherent potential is not static. Rather, potential increases for the young person who is well supported by their family, school, church, community and all levels of government. For many young people, peers are also an important aspect of their life. Benefits from stable peer relationships can significantly increase developmental outcomes. However, these same peer relationships can create tension for the young person and their family.

Developing the young person's potential helps to establish a good pathway that will assist to maximise achievements as an adult. Nurses have a significant role during these transitions, especially within the community, where most nursing and healthcare for this group occurs. The foundational support structure for the young person is the family, a source of strength and protection. A family-focused approach to nursing enhances the outcomes of healthcare for the young person. This chapter will address three keys strategies for promoting health and wellbeing and providing best nursing care to the young person:

1. developing the connections and relationships between nurses and the young person in partnerships
2. enabling the family and the young person in decision making, and
3. valuing and promoting family strengths.

Setting the scene: a clinical scenario

As an adolescent health nurse working in a rural community health centre, you receive a referral from the local high school. Becky, a 14-year-old female, is legally competent to give consent for her own healthcare and has accepted the referral (see Ch 4 for further information about informed consent and young people). Becky has been referred following noticeable behavioural changes that are negatively affecting her relationships with the teachers and other students. Her appearance has become increasingly 'scruffy' and her language has become nonchalant and at times offensive.

Becky has not previously been reported for disruptive behaviour at school. Becky was the highest achiever in Year 8 science last year. In primary school, Becky was the Year 6 representative on the student council. As a young child, Becky played well with all her friends and was an excellent mentor to the kindergarten children. She enjoyed visiting the nursing home through a local school community program, especially since her Nan was one of the residents. Shortly after Becky completed primary school, Nan passed away.

Becky lives with her mother Jill and older brother. Her parents divorced 2 years ago. She has not seen her father since, as he relocated interstate; yet, they speak on the telephone monthly. Becky used to enjoy talking to her mum after school; however, 3 months ago her mum re-entered the workforce taking a position as an evening waitress, involving long hours in the night and regular absence from home in the afternoon when Becky gets home. She misses sitting with her mum around the kitchen table. Her brother is also having trouble and Becky is worried that he may have started to take drugs. Last year he left school mid-year before completing Year 10 and has not had any employment since. He has stopped being home at teatime since mum started her new job and often returns home after mum finishes work. Becky's mum recently arranged a medical appointment for Becky to review her chronic yet usually controlled asthma following recent episodes of coughing at night.

Jill also mentioned to the general practitioner that Becky seemed unusually down. The medical notes identify that Becky has been neglecting to self-administer her asthma preventers and no formal diagnosis of any mental illness was made. This medical visit seemed to further upset Becky who is now saying to her mum 'everything is hopeless'. Becky continues to neglect to self-administer her preventers saying, 'What's the point? We all die of something.'

You spend time listening to Becky tell you her life story and start to develop a relationship with her. Becky starts by telling you 'things at home and school haven't been good this year and I've had some thoughts lately that are really scary. The thoughts started shortly after I broke up with my boyfriend. I don't like school any more and I take everything out on mum. I just don't know what to do anymore.' Becky asks, 'Can you help me cope please?' You also discover that she broke off with her boyfriend after her best friend started seeing him.

Becky's family and relationship losses and stress are affecting her. You ask Becky to draw a genogram, a diagram that depicts family relationships (Harris et al. 2006), and then you use this to identify important relationships in her life. Using the Australian Family Strengths Nursing Assessment Guide (see Table 1.2 in Ch 1), you start to explore with Becky her family's strengths. Since Becky is autonomous in seeking healthcare in this situation, you ask her how she would like your relationship to progress. You let Becky know that she is free to direct what her needs are and when she would like to meet with you. Becky decides that she would like to get together next week, and says she really liked talking to you about her life without being told what to do.

At your next visit, you further explore her family and personal strengths, and together you identify where Becky would like to be in 2 months time. Becky identifies that she wants to continue with her schooling and to make some new friends. She also wants to find some time to talk to her mum more—like she used to. Her brother's wellbeing is also a major concern, but just now she does not think she can deal too much with it, so you leave this for another day. A visit to her dad also seems a nice idea to her, perhaps in the summer holidays.

While reading this chapter, reflect on this scenario and consider how the issues discussed relate to Becky and your nursing. We will return to Becky at the end of this chapter.

Health and wellbeing of young people

Young childhood is often experienced as a period of delight and joy. This delight however can be interrupted with the onset of developmental changes that create challenges for the upper primary child and adolescent. The joys of childhood can be quickly forgotten when the tumultuous years of change appear. Despite community concerns over increasingly negative outcomes of late childhood and adolescence, statistics indicate that young people generally experience good health and succeed in their transition into young adulthood. Most young people in Australia are faring well. Mortality rates for all the major causes of death in children aged 1–14 in Australia continue to fall. The major cause of death in this age group remains injury and poisoning (Australian Institute of Health and Welfare 2005). Death rates for young people aged 12–24 also continue to fall, with the major cause in this age group also being injury and poisoning (Australian Institute of Health and Welfare 2003).

Yet, not every young person is doing so well. Too many young people experience traumatic periods in their adolescent years. Despite improvements in health statistics, in Australia, Aboriginal and Torres Straight Islander children and children from poorer socioeconomic backgrounds continue to experience higher mortality and morbidity rates, poorer developmental outcomes and generally reduced wellbeing when compared to other Australian children (Australian Institute of Health and Welfare 2005). Likewise, Maori and Pasifika children suffer from inequalities and injustices, which result in higher preventable mortality and morbidity rates than for non-Maori and non-Pasifika children (New Zealand Children's Commissioner 2006).

Statistics indicate that the intact family (where the child is the biological, adopted or foster child of both parents) remains the place where most young people live (Australian Institute of Health and Welfare 2005). Chapter 1 presented a detailed description of family characteristics in New Zealand and Australia. From data of families with children aged 4–12 years, the majority reported high levels of family cohesion, with cohesion higher generally in intact families than in lone-parent or blended families (Australian Institute of Health and Welfare 2005 p. 79). The resilience of the family to remain and to function well serves a protective function for children and young people. However, family and social changes (e.g. parental separation, divorce and relocation) can be impediments to the formation of secure relationships, and this may increase the risks to the health, wellbeing and actualisation of potential of the young person (Bronfenbrenner & Morris 1998, Eckersley 2001).

Some morbidity statistics continue to increase or remain high across a wide range of key indicators of health, development and wellbeing in young people in both Australia and New Zealand. Childhood obesity and type 2 diabetes are on the rise in both countries (Australian Institute of Health and Welfare 2005, New Zealand Children's Commissioner 2006). Adolescent alcohol abuse rates continue to increase (Hayes et al. 2004). Young people are responsible for more offences (judicial) than any other age group (Smart et al. 2003). Approximately 28% of young Australians are depressed, anxious, involved in antisocial behaviour and/or high alcohol consumption (Smart & Sanson 2005). Persistent struggles by Australian and New Zealand young people with abuse, homelessness, violence, teenage pregnancy, illicit drug usage, alcohol abuse, poor education outcomes, psychosocial disorders, depression and mental health are all problems facing young people and youth in recent years (McMurray 2007, Vimpani et al. 2002, New Zealand Children's Commissioner 2006). See Box 9.1 for the research basis of information about antisocial behaviour. These struggles may result in future trends of morbidity and mortality that we do not currently see. However, these recent patterns have significant bioecological factors that can be mediated with increased investment in primary healthcare and health promotion.

Box 9.1 Research highlight: patterns and precursors of adolescent antisocial behaviour

A longitudinal study undertaken by the Australian Institute of Family Studies in collaboration with Crime Prevention Victoria recruited 2443 children aged 4–8 months and their parents, who were a representative sample of Victoria. Through 13 annual or biannual waves of data, it has demonstrated that there were no direct links between the single factor of living in a disadvantaged location and antisocial behaviour. The research also found that the early adolescent years appear to be a crucial time of transition and for developing pathways towards antisocial behaviour.

Interventions aimed at late childhood and early adolescence are shown to successfully change negative pathways. Interventions that may be successful include developing personal skills in moderating difficult temperamental traits, improving relationships between adolescents and parents, assisting families to remain intact, assisting parents to develop parenting skills, and finding ways to enhance connectedness at school (Smart et al. 2003).

Illustrating the benefits of concerted health promotion to address issues confronting young people is the trend in young male suicide rates. In the early 1980s, the suicide rate for young Australian males aged 15–24 (19 per 100,000) was considerably lower than most other groups, yet by the late 1980s it had increased to the same rate as older males. The rate then peaked in 1997 at 31 per 100,000. Following public concerns and intensive injection of funds into prevention strategies, interventions and support for young men, the suicide rate has fallen dramatically back to 19 per 100,000 in 2001–02 (de Vass 2004).

Likewise, in New Zealand, youth suicide rates peaked in 1998 and have declined since (New Zealand Children's Commissioner 2006). Although the cause of the decline cannot be solely attributed to any one intervention, this illustrates the benefits gained through sound investment in health promotion and the huge cost we carry in loss of life and grief when primary healthcare strategies are neglected, especially for the young and vulnerable.

Effective health promotion that promotes youth resilience should have a bioecological focus. The greatest achievements in promoting health for the young person, especially the adolescent, can be gained through strengthening family cohesion and wellbeing. Other health promoting activities need to address broader bioecological factors. McMurray (2007 p. 199) identifies six major health issues affecting adolescents as:

1. mental and emotional health and maturity
2. physical health and wellbeing
3. minimisation of conditions that create risky behaviours
4. sustainable lifestyle habits
5. healthy environments, and
6. empowering structures and processes for successive generations.

The young person in context

Recent developmental research discoveries have indicated that genetic makeup does not solely determine human traits; rather, genetic messages interacting with environmental experiences determine developmental outcomes. Ecological factors affecting biological developments (such as parental interactions with their child impacting on early and young brain development) demonstrate how genetic endowment and environmental experiences interact to determine outcomes and human functioning (Vimpani 2001, Neill & Bowden 2004).

Genetic material contains blueprints for potential. However, they do not contain the processes. These processes of actualising genetic potential are found externally. Thus, development occurs through interactions between the individual and the environment (Rutter 2006). These interactions, which become effective if occurring regularly over time, are bi-directional. The ecology changes the person and the person changes the ecology. Therefore, the individual is active in their own development through selective patterns of attention, action and responses with people, objects and symbols.

Human interactions are the primary mechanism through which human genetic potential is actualised (Bronfenbrenner 2001). The bioecological theory of human development proposes that, by enhancing human interactions and environments, it is possible to increase the extent of genetic potential realised into development (Bronfenbrenner 2001, Bronfenbrenner & Ceci 1994 p. 568). The bioecological theory focuses on the mechanisms of development alongside the ecological context as equal determinants of development. This establishes the basis for understanding the young person within their environment as an active participant in their own development. It also establishes that in human development, the influential environment is not merely the immediate context in which the developing young person resides; rather, it also includes the interactions between people in various settings and the influences from larger surroundings. These are the bioecological determinants of development, health and wellbeing.

Understanding bioecological determinants assists nurses to promote optimal outcomes for the young person. Developing connections and relationships in partnership between the nurse, the young person and their family is a key strategy for nursing care of the young person. These connections are particularly important in promoting adolescent health and wellbeing, as they recognise the autonomy of the adolescent and promote partnerships between the adolescent and their nurse. Across all stages of life, nurses provide an important human input into the life, wellbeing, health and development of others. Understanding your role in the life of a young person and their family is necessary to enhance connectedness, facilitate communication and maximise empowerment.

In an empowering relationship, the nurse uses their power (skills, knowledge and will) for the other and rejects using power to control others (Balswick et al. 2005). Bioecological determinants can be grouped within three domains: the individual, the family and the community. Structuring nursing support across all three domains to enhance strengths will maximise health and development outcomes for the young person through supporting both their own and their family's resilience. Family resilience is defined as a family's healthy response and successful adaptation to the risks, stresses, adversities, everyday normality and changes of life, family and its members' experience (Smith 2002). The enhanced health and development outcomes influence the individual, family and the community strengths, thus creating a positive cycle in the bioecological determinants (see Fig 9.1).

Figure 9.1 The resilience cycle

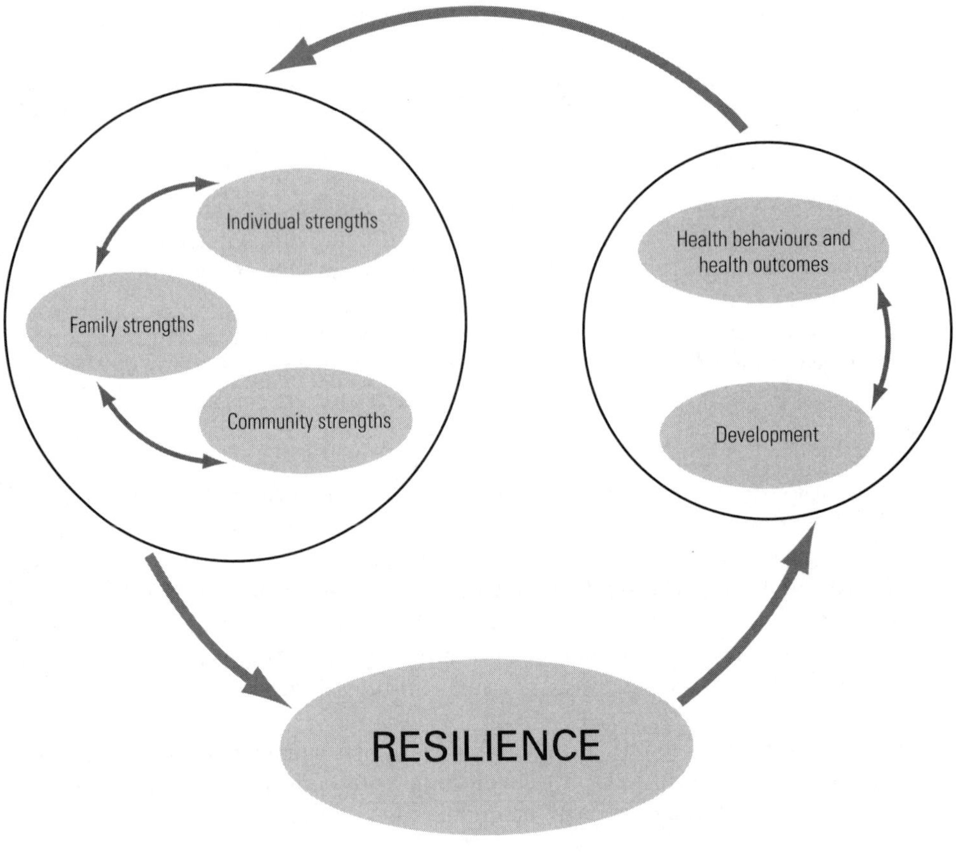

Protective and risk factors for young people

Determining risk is a central task of population health research. Risk in this research means 'the probability that an event will occur' (Young 2005 p. 177). Risk is commonly conceived of as the likelihood of a negative outcome rather than the likelihood of a positive one. To clarify this concept, protective factors increase the likelihood of a positive outcome and risk factors increase the likelihood of a negative outcome. Population health researchers undertake analysis of a phenomenon (the risk or protective factor) at the level of the whole population. Other health research undertaken at the individual or small group level is applied health research. Applied health research contributes towards understanding and testing the findings from population health research and broadens the understanding of health and illness through a lens of human values (Young 2005). From population health research we can identify protective and risk factors, and from applied health research we can understand why these factors occur and what contributes to or hinders their occurrence.

Many health and wellbeing outcomes are identified to be amendable to various risk and protective factors (Wilkinson & Marmot 2003). Both risk and protective factors are likely to be cumulative—that is, the greater the protective factors and the less the risk factors, resilience is enhanced and outcomes are maximised (Blum & Ireland 2004). A risk-focused approach identifies problems or trouble in an endeavour to isolate what went wrong and the negative consequences of the various actions, failures or breakdowns. Findings from troubled families demonstrate the scope of the challenge that some young people face (Beautrais 2000, Bond et al. 2000, Blum & Nelson-Mmari 2004). As a result, nursing care and health promotion tend to emphasise treating young people and families with identifiable risks, highlighting negative attitudes, eliminating behaviours related to risk, and warning those not already engaged in the risky behaviour.

Risk-focused research findings provide little guidance about what young people and families can do to optimise positive outcomes. Risk-reduction approaches to health promotion do not appear to be effective and risk-focused deficit models should change to strengths models (Blum 1998 p. 373). Exploring protective factors provides a basis to structure health promotion and nursing care of young people, while not neglecting the risk factors that young people face (Blum et al. 2002). See Table 1.1 in Chapter 1 for a list of individual, family and community risk and protective factors that influence early childhood health, and see Table 10.2 in Chapter 10 for risk and protective factors for psychopathology in children and young people.

The identification of risk, however, is not without criticism. Some risks may be modified through ecological factors that negate the risk for some yet not for others. These modifying factors are often unknown. Placing restrictions on people's behaviours because of the identified risk, based on assumptions that may not be generalisable, is problematic. Even after extended exposure to severe negative experiences, children demonstrate variations in their long-term outcomes (Wise 2003). Resnick et al. (1997) identified that:

> '. . . some children who are at high risk of health compromising behaviours negotiate adolescence, avoiding behaviours that predispose them to negative

health outcomes, while others relatively advantaged socially and economically, sustain significant morbidity as a consequence of their behaviour'.

At other times, risks that have demonstrated a weak correlation in population health research may indeed pose a severe risk to certain susceptible individuals or groups. The decision to identify a risk as being undesirable is constructed through social, cultural and political processes, which are disempowering to the individual and allows health administrators to allocate blame to the victim based on their association with the risk (Patterson & Lupton 1996). Risk findings tend to categorise groups of people as 'problems', without any effort to understand the individuals within these groups (Lupton 1999). For example, being an adolescent is often seen as a risk itself, one that is resolved by obtaining the status of an adult.

Although it is known that protective factors can modify the effects of risk factors and generate wellbeing, the ways in which various protective factors and risk factors interact to protect young people from engaging in risk-taking behaviour and enhance health and development is not known (Wise 2003, Smart et al. 2003).

Clinical focus for nursing the young person

With the advent of modern nursing from the late 1800s and the rise of the medical profession during the 1900s, nursing practice became increasingly dominated by a biomedical approach with its reductionist and deficit focus (Wearing 2004). Nursing has predominantly been understood as one person caring for another person, with most nurses considering the individual as the boundary of their care (Segaric & Hall 2005).

This creates two problems. Firstly, in caring for the young person, the family is viewed in terms of their potential contribution towards the present illness instead of their contributions towards wellness (Darbyshire 1994). Secondly, the family becomes excluded from both decision making and contributing towards care because the nurse–client relationship becomes the dominant relationship. In this relationship, the nurse becomes the expert, who possesses the solutions and controls the resources (Wynaden et al. 2006, Griffin 2003). In other words, the biomedical orientation of clinical nursing decreases the centrality of the family, which leads the nurse to fail to appreciate the importance of the family to health outcomes. In short, a biomedical model unwittingly prepares nurses to overlook the family.

The negative effect of alienating young people from their parents during hospitalisation was established by 1970, yet few changes were seen until the early 1990s (Middleton 2005). Attitudes towards the care of the young person have now changed. Nursing care of the young person has become inclusive of families, with models of nursing care such as family-centred care introduced on an increasing scale (Young et al. 2006). Now nursing care of the young person emphasises the relationships, connections and the partnership between the family and the nurse. Nursing care of the young person attempts to enable the family and the young person in their decision making related to healthcare. While enabling the family in this process, the nurse needs to remain aware of the struggle for autonomy that the young person is attempting to manage, while they are needing support from their loved ones when faced with health issues. More recent advancement in nursing the young person sees nursing displaying a family-strengths focus. These developments are critical for the optimising of community-based and primary healthcare of young people.

Nurses developing connections and enabling relationships

Developing connections and relationships between nurses and the young person in partnerships is one of the keys to providing best nursing care of the young person. If you review the clinical scenario at the beginning of the chapter, you will notice this approach. Crole and Smith (2002) highlighted four important phases in developing the relationship between nurses and the young person.

Initially, during the *introductory phase*, the young person and their family may make the initial connection with their nurse, especially in a community setting such as a school or community health service. At other times, nurses make the initial contact with the young person. Nonetheless, strategies nurses use to assist in establishing common bonds with the young person include talking about television shows and participating in favourite activities. These times give an opportunity to participate in conversations that demonstrate how the nurse values the young person, without the pressure of them having to comply with any requests or undergo any procedures. Establishing a good rapport with the young person allays anxiety and may help avert adverse behaviour (Mills 2005).

Once the relationship has commenced, it is important to *build trust*. Nurses' use of age-appropriate language, social activities, providing explanations, allowing participation in decision making and goal setting, encouragement and adequate preparation for procedures all help build trust in the relationship. A young person will be more trusting of nurses who are willing to get down on their level and interact on their terms. Social interactions have many benefits for both the young person and nurse. It is a normalising experience for the young person (Hall & Reit 2000).

Often nurses are required to make decisions that challenge the connection that has developed in the relationship with the young person. During the *decision-making phase*, nurses need to decide how much control is given to the young person. Giving the young person some control is a common technique nurses use to enable the young person once trust is established. In general, there are no guidelines that regulate nurses delegating self-care tasks and enabling the young person to participate in the decision-making process. Issues of informed consent and working within the scope of practice should be articulated within the employer's policy and procedures manual and may determine appropriate actions in some situations. These decisions are complicated when the young person is estranged from their parents or hesitant to include them in the decision. When promoting lifestyle choices in health promotion activities, an enabling approach facilitates empowerment and significantly increases the likelihood of long-term benefits being achieved.

At times during the relationship, the young person may see their nurse whom they trusted as responsible for the discomfort and pain experienced. *Comforting and reassuring* the young person assists to maintain or re-establish the trusting relationship. Techniques such as praising the young person for their courage to address their challenges and getting the young person to consider what they have achieved towards their goals help restore the young person's trust and build their self-esteem.

The four phases of the relationship between nurses and the young person, as illustrated in Figure 9.2, highlight the importance of building every stage of the relationship and the interconnectivity of each stage. If trust is not established or is impeded throughout the four phases, it becomes difficult to gain the young person's cooperation or deliver optimal nursing care. Nurses need to move between these four relationship phases to skilfully optimise the outcomes from nursing encounters with the young person. Nurses become engaged in the lives of the young person and the family to help them cope with the difficulties they face. This engagement requires commitment and involvement, yet finding the right level of involvement is necessary in achieving a therapeutic long-term relationship (Hawes 2005).

Figure 9.2 The four phases of the nurse–young person relationship

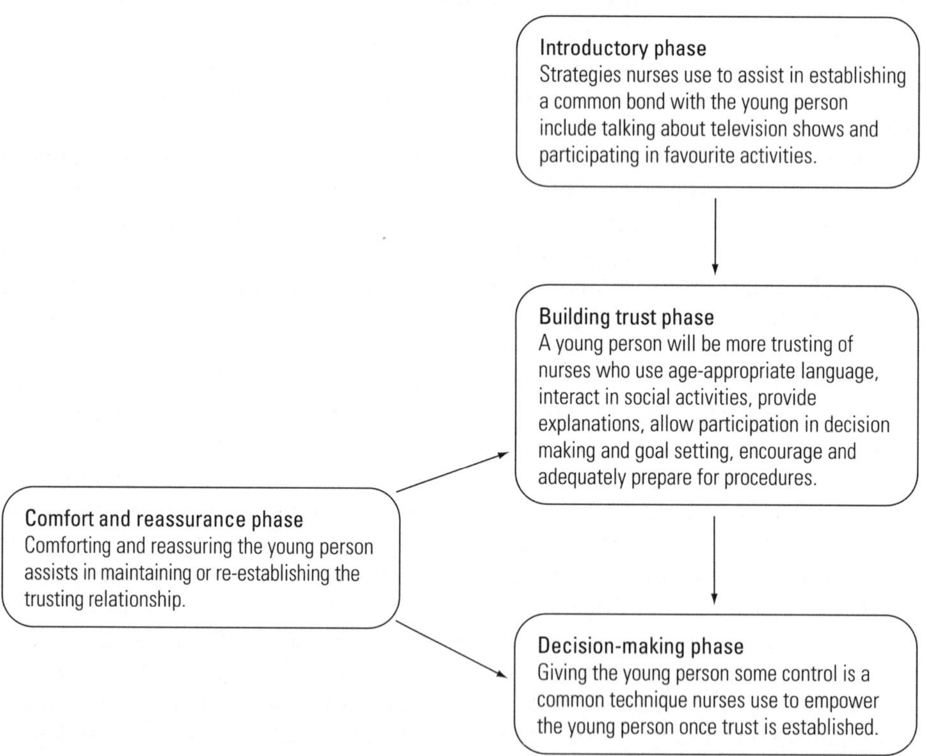

Source: Adapted from N Crole and L Smith 2002 Examining the phases of nursing care of the hospitalised child. *Australian Nursing Journal* 9(8):30–1.

Valuing and assessing family strengths with the young person

The strengths perspective (see Ch 1) lends itself particularly well to nursing young people. All young people have strengths that nurses can draw on through primary healthcare and health promotion activities. There is emerging strong evidence for the importance of nurses caring for the young person to help families develop strengths. Overwhelmingly, researchers and health advocates conclude that strong families assist young people to develop resilience, help overcome life challenges and crises, and develop enhanced health and wellbeing outcomes (Denham 2003, Joronen & Astedt-Kurki 2005, Wolkow & Ferguson 2001, Wertlieb 2003).

Young people often feel disconnected from their family and some are alienated. Parents often feel despondent, worn out and challenged by the transitions and choices of the young person. It is most important for nurses to help young people identify their place in their family, as well as helping families identify their functioning (past and present) strengths and facilitate their further development. If you review the clinical scenario at the beginning of the chapter, you will notice this approach. Helping young people to be more aware of their connectedness to their family enhances their self-esteem and resilience. The young person should be explicitly asked to identify their family strengths. Identifying and documenting a history of family strengths can act as a significant means of helping the young person and their family draw on their strengths during stressful times (Sittner et al. 2005, Feeley & Gottlieb 2000).

Identifying their family strengths can also be a means of developing good connections with the young person. When a positive and encouraging perspective in their nurse is recognised, their optimism in the outcomes will increase. Adopting a positive perception of adversity inspires and encourages the young person to know that they have the strength to be resilient, to withstand stressors and to recognise that growth occurs from experiencing stressful conditions and transitions. Try the activity set out in Box 9.2.

Box 9.2 Critical reflections: assessing family strengths and the young person

Utilising the Australian Family Strengths Nursing Assessment Guide found in Chapter 1, Table 1.2, engage in a conversation with a young person who you know about their family's strengths and how their family functions across the eight qualities. Explore what goals the young person is currently striving towards concerning their health, wellbeing and family. You can use the clinical scenario with Becky as a guide to this activity.

Nurses relating to the young person with challenging behaviour

Nurses can be confronted by a range of behaviours in the young person, which may be perceived as challenging (Russell et al. 2003). These may include behaviours considered normal while the young person is experiencing transitions in development, to those that are aggressive, threatening and overtly risky. Some challenging behaviours displayed by the young person may be associated with specific diagnoses impacting on self-control and development, such as autism and hyperactive and attention disorders. Some challenging behaviours may be associated with communication or with a family's perceived lack of interest in the young person's welfare.

At times, the family may abdicate their involvement in the care of a young person displaying challenging behaviour, effectively leaving the nurse to negotiate directly with the young person. Even when the young person and the family are empowered to participate in the decision making and nursing care, they may still decide not to adopt the path suggested or encouraged by the nurse.

A recent grounded theory study of paediatric nurses asked participants to define challenging behaviours, as they perceived them, in 7–14 year olds (Wood 2003). In this study, physical aggression and violence were identified as the most challenging to nurses, particularly when the behaviour was unexpected and essential care had to be provided. Despite the difficulties experienced by nurses when confronted with challenging behaviour, caring for the young person is often both stimulating and satisfying.

Now returning to Becky from our clinical scenario, we can see how important it is that the connections she has in her life are further strengthened. Her connections with her parents, her brother, her friends and her school have been challenged recently. Through a family-strengths perspective, these challenges and stresses can be reframed as transitions that are leading to growth in the relationships. It is through enhancing the strengths in Becky's life across all areas (individual, family and community, as shown in the resilience cycle in Fig 9.1) that resilience is strengthened and her health and wellbeing outcomes are protected and enhanced.

Further challenges that Becky may encounter associated with adolescence include her sexuality and sexual behaviour, her body image and self-esteem, along with being resistant to the misuse of drugs and alcohol. Becky's concerns for her brother are real and will need exploring. What actions Becky should and could take are dependent on many factors not identified within this scenario. For now, ensuring Becky feels connected to her family, friends and community is the highest priority.

Conclusion

Nursing of the young person can incorporate a strengths perspective as a basis of nursing care. Understanding of influences on health and development has shifted from a predisposing medicalised focus to a broad understanding of bioecological determinates. Nursing actions and attitudes that enable the young person and the family, build connections and relationships, and help mobilise strengths, are the most effective nursing strategies for enhancing health and development. Nurses increase connectedness to the young person through spending time developing a relationship with the young person, talking about things that matter to them, and including the young person and the family in the decision-making process as much as they are able and willing.

Practice tips

Nurses caring for the young person from a family-strengths perspective will seek to:

» look for healthy intentions in the young person and in their family
» support the young person's courage in taking actions towards their desired goals
» assess operational strengths that can be encouraged
» seek to maintain the family's functioning and coherence

» attempt to collaborate with the whole family in a partnership
» enable the young person and their family through active participation in decision making whenever appropriate (as determined by the young person and the family) and if possible (ensuring negotiation and safe preparation and education has occurred), and
» relate to the young person directly through building connections at an age-appropriate level.

Useful resources

Australian Government Department of Families, Community Services and Indigenous Affairs—Youth: www.facs.gov.au/internet/facsinternet.nsf/youth/nav.htm.
Australian Institute of Health and Welfare (AIHW) *Health inequalities monitoring series*. Available at www.aihw.gov.au/publications/index.cfm/series/240.
Centre for Adolescent Health: www.rch.org.au/cah/index.cfm?doc_id=833.
Children, Youth and Family Consortium: www.cyfc.umn.edu/welcome.html.
Families First—Better Futures: www.familiesfirst.nsw.gov.au/public/s42_strategy_FF/strategies.aspx?id=2.
The spirit of generation Y. Young people, spirituality and society: http://dlibrary.acu.edu.au/research/ccls/spir/sppub/sppub.htm.
UNL for families: http://unlforfamilies.unl.edu/Index.htm.
Victorian Adolescent Health Cohort Study *2000 stories*: www.mcri.edu.au/pages/2000-stories/.

References

Australian Institute of Health and Welfare (AIHW) 2003 *Australia's young people: their health and wellbeing*. Cat. No. PHE50. AIHW, Canberra.
Australian Institute of Health and Welfare (AIHW) 2005 *A picture of Australia's children*. Cat. No. PHE58. AIHW, Canberra.
Balswick J, King P, Reimer K 2005 *The reciprocating self. Human development in theological perspective*. InterVarsity Press, Illinois.
Beautrais AL 2000 Risk factors for suicide and attempted suicide among young people. *Australian and New Zealand Journal of Psychiatry* 34:420–36.
Blum R 1998 Healthy youth development as a model for youth health promotion: A review. *Journal of Adolescent Health* 22:368–75.
Blum R, Ireland M 2004 Reducing risk, increasing protective factors: findings from the Caribbean Youth Health Survey. *Journal of Adolescent Health* 35:493–500.
Blum R, McNeely C, Nonnemaker J 2002 Vulnerability, risk and protection. *Journal of Adolescent Health* 31(S):28–39.
Blum R, Nelson-Mmari K 2004 The health of young people in a global context. *Journal of Adolescent Health* 35:402–18.
Bond L, Thomas L, Toumbourou J et al. 2000 *Improving the lives of young Victorians in our community: a survey of risk and protective factors*. Centre for Adolescent Health, Melbourne.

Bronfenbrenner U 2001 The bioecological theory of human development. Article 1 in U Bronfenbrenner (ed.) 2005, *Making human beings human: biological perspectives on human development*. Sage, Thousand Oaks, California.

Bronfenbrenner U, Ceci S 1994 Nature–nurture reconceptualized in developmental perspective: a bioecological model. *Psychological Review* 101(4):568–86.

Bronfenbrenner U, Morris P 1998 The bioecological model of human development. In L Damon & R Lerner (eds) 2006, *Handbook of child psychology*, 6th ed, Vol. 1, R Lerner (ed.) *Theoretical models of human development*. John Wiley, Hoboken, New Jersey, pp. 795–829.

Crole N, Smith L 2002 Examining the phases of nursing care of the hospitalised child. *Australian Nursing Journal* 9(8):30–1.

Darbyshire P 1994 *Living with a sick child in hospital: the experiences of parents and nurses*. Chapman & Hall, Melbourne.

Denham S 2003 *Family health. A framework for nursing*. FA Davis, Philadelphia.

de Vass D 2004 *Diversity and change in Australian families: statistical profiles*. Australian Institute of Family Studies, Melbourne.

Eckersley R 2001 Culture, health and well-being. In R Eckersley, J Dixson & B Douglas (eds), *The social origins of health and well-being*. Cambridge University Press, Melbourne.

Feeley N, Gottlieb L 2000 Nursing approaches for working with family strengths and resources. *Journal of Family Nursing* 6(1):9–24.

Griffin T 2003 Facing challenges to family-centered care II: anger in the clinical setting. *Pediatric Nursing* 29(3):212–14.

Hall C, Reit M 2000 Enhancing the state of play in children's nursing. *Journal of Child Health Care* 4(2):49–54.

Harris P, Nagy S, Vardaxis N 2006 *Mosby's dictionary of medicine, nursing and health professions*. Elsevier, Sydney.

Hawes R 2005 Therapeutic relationships with children and families. *Pediatric Nursing* 17(6):15–18.

Hayes L, Smart D, Toumbourou J, Sanson A 2004 *Parental influences on adolescent alcohol use*, Research Report No. 10. Australian Institute of Family Studies, Melbourne.

Joronen K, Astedt-Kurki P 2005 Familial contribution to adolescent subjective well-being. *International Journal of Nursing Practice* 11:125–33.

Lupton D 1999 *Risk*. Routledge, London.

McMurray A 2007 *Community health and wellness. A socioecological approach*, 3rd edn. Elsevier, Sydney.

Middleton C 2005 A short journey down a long road: the emergence of professional bodies. In A Sidey & D Widdas (eds), *Textbook of community children's nursing*, 2nd edn. Elsevier, Edinburgh.

Mills D 2005 Play therapy within community children's nursing. In A Sidey & D Widdas (eds), *Textbook of community children's nursing*, 2nd edn. Elsevier, Edinburgh.

Neill S, Bowden L 2004 Central nervous system development. In S Neill & H Knowles (eds), *The biology of child health: a reader in development and assessment*. Palgrave, Hampshire.

New Zealand Children's Commissioner 2006 *More than an apple a day: children's right to good health*. Office of the Children's Commissioner, Wellington, New Zealand.

Patterson A, Lupton D 1996 *The new public health: health and self in the age of risk.* Allen & Unwin, Sydney.

Resnick MD, Bearman PS, Blum RW et al. 1997 Protecting adolescents from harm. Findings from the national longitudinal study on adolescent health. *Journal of the American Medical Association* 278(10):823–32.

Russell S, Daly J, Hughs E, Op't Hoog C 2003 Nurses and 'difficult' patients: negotiating non-compliance. *Journal of Advanced Nursing* 43(3):281–7.

Rutter M 2006 *Genes and behavior: nature–nurture interplay explained.* Blackwell, Oxford, UK.

Segaric C, Hall W 2005 The family theory–practice gap: a matter of clarity? *Nursing Inquiry* 12(3):210–18.

Sittner B, DeFrain J, Hudson D 2005 Effects of high risk pregnancies on families. *American Journal of Maternal Child Nursing* 30(2):121–6.

Smart D, Sanson A 2005 What is life like for young Australians and how well are they faring? *Family Matters* 70:46–53.

Smart D, Vassallo S, Sanson A et al. 2003 *Patterns and precursors of adolescent antisocial behaviour. Types, resiliency and environmental influences*, Second Report. Crime Prevention Victoria, Melbourne.

Smith L 2002 Caring for the family. *Australian Nursing Journal* 10(1):CU1-2.

Vimpani G 2001 Health inequalities: the seeds are sown in childhood, what about remedies? In R Eckersley, J Dixson & B Douglas (eds), *The social origins of health and well-being*. Cambridge University Press, Melbourne.

Vimpani G, Patton G, Hayes A 2002 The relevance of child and adolescent development for outcomes in education, health and life success. In A Sanson (ed.), *Children's health and development: new research directions for Australia*, AIFS Research Report No. 8. Australian Institute of Family Studies, Melbourne.

Wearing M 2004 Medical dominance and the division of labour in the health professions. In C Grbich (ed.), *Health in Australia. Sociological concepts and issues*, 3rd edn. Pearson, Sydney.

Wertlieb D 2003 Converging trends in family research and pediatrics: recent findings for the American Academy of Pediatrics task force on the family. *Pediatrics* 111(6):1572–87.

Wilkinson R, Marmot M 2003 *Social determinants of health: the solid facts*, 2nd edn. World Health Organization Regional Office for Europe, Copenhagen, Denmark. Available at www.euro.who.int/document/e81384.pdf.

Wise S 2003 *Family structure, child outcomes and environmental mediators. An overview of the development in diverse families study*, Research Paper No. 30. Australian Institute of Family Studies, Melbourne.

Wolkow K, Ferguson H 2001 Community factors in the development of resiliency: considerations and future directions. *Community Mental Health Journal* 37(6):489–98.

Wood B, 2003 *Paediatric nurses' definitions of and responses to challenging behaviour in 7–14 year old children on the paediatric ward: a grounded theory study.* Unpublished thesis Bachelor of Nursing (Honours), University of Tasmania, (supervised by L Smith).

Wynaden D, Ladzinski U, Lapsley J et al. 2006 The care giving experience: how much do health professionals understand? *Collegian* 13(3):6–10.

Young J, McCann D, Watson K et al. 2006 Negotiation for care for a hospitalised child: parental perspective. *Neonatal, Paediatric and Child Health Nursing* 9(2):4–13.

Young TK 2005 *Population health. Concepts and methods*, 2nd edn. Oxford University Press, New York.

Chapter 10

Promoting mental health

Margaret McAllister and Christine Handley

Learning outcomes

Reading this chapter will help you to:

» understand the reasons for the need to equally emphasise prevention, treatment and promotion in mental health work

» understand how knowledge of developmental stages assists in shaping interventions that serve to promote mental health in young people and their families

» identify the range of mental health strategies clinicians use within the spectrum of interventions for mental disorders

» describe day-to-day practice activities useful in promoting a young person's mental health and wellbeing, and

» discuss issues important to organisational planning so that services in which you work can build their capacity to provide youth-centred care.

Introduction

In this chapter, we discuss the issue of youth mental health and outline strategies for promoting mental health and wellbeing. As a nurse, you may be working with children and/or adolescents as a specialist CAMHS (Child and Adolescent Mental Health Services) nurse. Alternatively, you may be working with young people in a school setting, in child and family services, in a general practice setting, in a community health centre or as a youth worker with young children who are homeless and living on the streets. You may be a nurse working in a mental health or youth justice residential setting. The young people with whom you work may live in urban, rural or primarily Indigenous communities. The principles of mental health promotion are applicable across all of these different work settings.

We tell a story of a vulnerable adolescent whose experiences flow on to affect the health and wellbeing of her family and, without effective intervention, would be likely to interrupt her relationships and achievements at school, with peers and on into the future. As authors we have attempted to model a *person-centred* approach to thinking about and working with the young person, as this is a key feature and aim for practice development. We have also included discussion on both *knowledge* and *practice* issues, because the development of theoretical understanding and education, as well as practical skills and strategies, are two essential ingredients for change.

Setting the scene: a clinical scenario

The nurse

Imagine you are a postgraduate nursing student who has only recently commenced employment for the first time in a Child and Adolescent Mental Health Centre. You are sitting in on a referral interview for the purposes of assessment. Present is a 13-year-old girl, Chelsea, and her mother, Vicki. Chelsea appears unhappy, angry and uncommunicative. She scowls at you and her mother and gives every indication that she is not happy at all about being here. During the interview, Vicki is critical of her daughter's behaviour towards her of late and she tells you that her daughter is saying that she wants to die and hates her mother.

Chelsea

Now imagine yourself as a 13-year-old girl who lives with her mum and her younger sister and an older brother. Your mother is always yelling at you and you are convinced that she hates you. Your older brother is a 'weirdo' and does horrible things to everyone at home. Your younger sister is a 'pain', shares your bedroom and is always touching your stuff. You never have any peace at home. You feel like life is not worth living and write notes to your mother telling her you want to die. You hate school because you are being bullied by an older girl and no one seems to take this seriously. You feel powerless to deal with this on your own. You feel very angry with your family and you hate the world. Nothing good ever happens to you and there is nothing to look forward to.

This scenario, which we return to later in the chapter, represents a typical referral of a young person to a mental health facility. Chelsea and young people like her could be referred by a general practitioner, a paediatrician, a school guidance counsellor or a community nurse. It would be very easy to focus solely on the presenting problems and not see Chelsea as a whole person capable of overcoming the difficulties she is experiencing in her life. Initial energies by the nurse might be directed towards making a clinical diagnosis and treating the identified problem. However, this would be quite unproductive for both Chelsea and her family. Why? How are the concepts of mental health prevention, early intervention and promotion relevant to Chelsea's situation? Think about the usefulness and limitations of diagnosis within a mental health promotion context. What can you do as a nurse to ensure that prevention and early intervention initiatives are undertaken in your workplace?

Mental health issues in Australia and New Zealand

It is important to be clear about what mental health and mental disorder actually mean, because the way an issue is conceptualised can influences the ways it is prevented and responded to. The term 'mental illness' is an ill-fitting descriptor. It is really a metaphor for describing dysfunction. Very few mental health problems can be confidently attributed to physical abnormalities and thus they are not illnesses in the true sense. So too, biological treatments are likely to treat only the symptoms of disorder and do little to promote health and wellbeing in the long term, and do nothing to prevent disorders. Thus, it is important to search for a definition that reaches beyond a biological understanding of mental health and disorder.

Freud, for example, defined mental health simply as the ability to love, work and play. Almost 70 years later, the World Health Organization (2001) describes it similarly. Positive mental health is a:

> '. . . state of wellbeing in which the individual realises his or her own abilities, can cope with the normal stresses of life, can work productively and fruitfully, and is able to make a contribution to his or her community'.

In both definitions, the emphasis is on having a rich internal, imaginative and creative life, and the ability to relate with others and engage competently in meaningful activities.

In order to be able to understand the issue of mental health promotion within Australia and New Zealand, it is important to be aware of the extent of the problem that mental disorder creates for individuals and groups. One in five (20%) Australians and New Zealanders will have a mental health problem at some stage in their lifetime, and these primarily develop because of noxious life events such as experiencing violence or stress. Up to 2% will develop serious mental disorders, such as schizophrenia or bipolar affective disorder, and these tend to develop during adolescence or early adulthood. According to Mindframe (n.d.), a media resource supported by the Australian mental health strategy, 14% of Australian children and young people aged 4–17 have mental health problems.

This rate of mental health problems is found in all age and gender groups. Boys are slightly more likely to experience mental health problems than girls. Also, there is a higher prevalence of child and adolescent mental health problems among those living in low-income, step/blended and sole-parent families (Sawyer et al. 2000). This means that, each year, about half a million Australian and 115,000 New Zealand youth are affected and will suffer from at least one mental illness episode. Only a quarter of those needing help will receive it.

Certain groups of children and young people are more vulnerable and have particular needs, including but not exclusive to:

- Aboriginal and Torres Strait Islander and Maori children and young people
- children and young people in rural and remote communities
- children and young people separated from their families
- homeless children and young people
- children and young people affected by adverse life events, and
- children with health, developmental or learning problems.

Despite ongoing research, the causes of these illnesses remain poorly understood, and so it is still not possible to accurately predict or prevent their onset. People still lack timely access to services, and many consumers criticise healthcare providers for being patronising or stigmatising (SANE Australia 2004) leading to feelings of isolation or discrimination. Furthermore, most services still tend to be oriented to mature adults who have disability secondary to mental health problems. This makes recovery and adaptation to illness delayed and thus disability and all of its associated costs are increased.

However, alternative approaches are appearing and are highlighted throughout this chapter. One example is Vibe, a New Zealand community action network (see Box 10.1). It is open to young adults in Auckland with experience of mental distress and a passion for positive social change. It was created in 2002 'by youth for youth' and has as its touchstones 'Youth; Connection; Hope; Growth; Uniqueness; Diversity; Respect and Creativity'. Vibe has an action-oriented focus and implements projects in the youth community that reduce discrimination by and towards youth around experiences of mental distress.

Box 10.1 Practice highlight: Vibe online

For information about Vibe, you can go to New Zealand's mental health promotion and prevention newsletter at www.mindnet.org.nz. This link also allows you to access the Mental Health Foundation of New Zealand, which provides a wealth of mental health information and resources, including demographic information and services for young people in New Zealand. The foundation defines mental health promotion as work to enable individuals, whanau, organisations and communities to improve and sustain their mental health and realise their full potential (www.mentalhealth.org.nz).

The need for better mental health promotion and illness prevention

In 1992, following a Royal Commission into the human rights of people with mental illness, the Australian Health Ministers recognised the need to work together and move beyond state boundaries to improve conditions and services for people with mental health problems. A collaborative framework for national reform was established, the National Mental Health Strategy, and a number of important changes have occurred, including prioritising mental health prevention and promotion. New Zealand had a similar experience, with the 1996 Mason Inquiry that led to the establishment of a national Mental Health Commission (1998). Australian and New Zealand clinicians now draw on the US-based Institute of Medicine's spectrum of interventions model of mental health service delivery (Mrazek & Haggerty 1994). This model (see Fig 10.1) emphasises not just the treatment of disorders, but also prevention, treatment, recovery and health promotion.

Nurses working in mental health

In essence, the nurse's role in mental health is to support the restoration of mental health and wellbeing for individuals and families using skilled, professional care. As

Figure 10.1 Spectrum of interventions

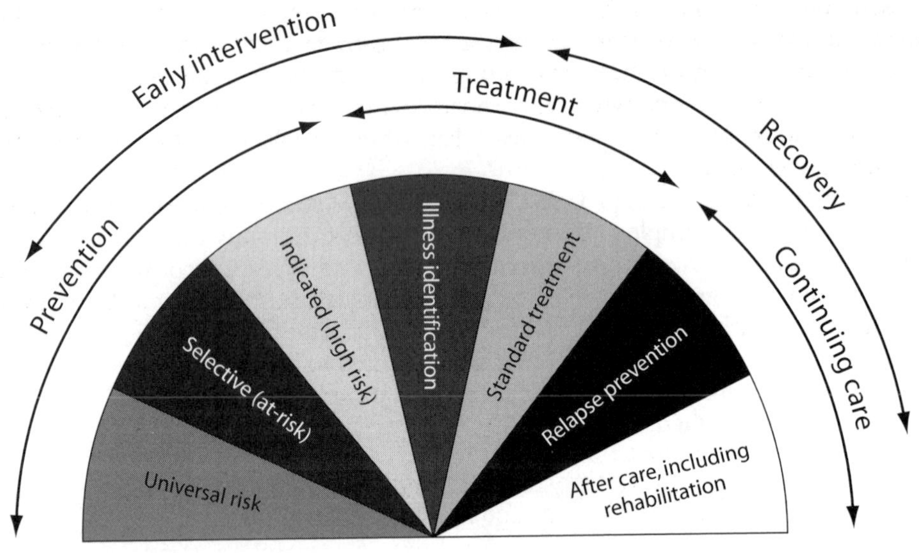

Source: P Mrazek and R Haggerty R (eds) 1994 *Reducing risks for mental disorders: frontiers for intervention research.* National Academy Press, Washington DC.

mentioned in the introduction to the chapter, nurses with child and youth mental health skills are located in various contexts throughout the community, including the large women's health units where infant mental health nurses can be found, schools, community health centres, hospitals, and specialised services such as drug and alcohol centres and recovery programs.

Nursing care is provided in a range of ways: by educating the public so that they understand mental health and replace any stereotypes with accurate knowledge; by cultivating a trusting relationship in which mental health problems can be explored and understood; by encouraging people to adhere to treatments such as medications and cognitive behavioural training; by conveying hope so that the person finds meaning in the experience, develops strengths and makes social connections; and by motivating people to make good use of future services and continue therapeutic work (Happell et al. 2002). Even though there are many outstanding, dedicated and professional mental health nurses, in any system there is room for improvement and, in mental health, there are some issues that are in need of practice development.

Some critics have suggested that mental health is hampered by poor interprofessional understanding and this has led to fragmentation of care (Carradice & Round 2004). (See Ch 2 for a discussion of silo culture in health programs.) When hospital services fail to communicate effectively with community services, clients may not be followed up in a timely way and adherence to treatments may diminish (Wright & Cummings 2005). Clinicians may sometimes feel unfulfilled because they lack knowledge and skills that help them be focused and strategic with clients (Bowles et al. 2001).

Solutions to these problems rest in a combination of additional funding for increased staff, improved educational preparation and access to continuing education and training, and introduction of models of care that move beyond a problem-orientation towards a strengths and recovery model (see the practice highlight in Box 10.2). Studies have shown that these changes do produce positive effects, not just for the nurses themselves, but also in better patient outcomes (Aspinwall & Staudinger 2003). For example, Webb (2002) found that clinicians who respond with empathy, a non-judgmental stance and supportive counselling skills have a positive effect on outcomes for young clients. These clients are more likely to stay for treatment, to use the health service again rather than attempt to inadequately self-manage and to have organised follow-up care. At the cultural level, where communities offer sources for self-esteem, a sense of purpose, support from parents, family and community, suicides are reduced and wellbeing is enhanced (Resnick et al. 1997).

Box 10.2 Practice highlight: a solution-focused approach

Taking a problem-centred focus is particularly unhelpful when working with young people because, by its nature, a problem orientation tends to search for what's going wrong with a person, and usually involves an expert applying solutions. This can compound loss of hope and be disempowering. How to be solution-focused with young people remains a challenge. A group of Australian youth health workers (Stacey et al. 2002) collated their strategies. We add to these some practical ideas for application and offer these practical approaches:

- Respect young people as knowledgeable. Ask the person to talk about the ways they cope with present and past challenges.
- Go beyond seeing young people as objects or people at risk. They have strengths and resilience. Use an assessment framework that allows you to understand more than the person's presenting problem. Make an effort to get to know their talents, gifts, hobbies, dreams and goals.
- Facilitate trust and listen with genuineness. Being trustworthy, reliable, respectful and honourable, even if you do not have the answers or if you make a mistake, are ways for you to show your merit as a caring person.
- Try to see solutions instead of just the problem. Look for presenting problems or issues and then work with the person to set realistic goals to solve each issue. Be solution focused, but not solution forced.
- Focus on exceptions to the problem-laden story so you can use those exceptions to build solutions and build optimism and hope. For example, you could ask, 'Do you remember a time when you felt closer with your mother and family. What were you all doing at that time? Tell me more about those times.' Then, you can discuss the kinds of qualities the person conveyed that perhaps might be useful to harness and develop in the present time.
- Involve young people in aspects of the service. For example, young people could be in charge of planning special education events, or for creating resources to promote the service to other young people.
- Attempt to find meaning during all social interactions. Sometimes interactions can be educative and enlightening, rather than always simply fun or a distraction. For example, if you go to the cinema, spend time discussing the strong characters in the movie and help the person identify with the pro-social behaviours.

Developmental stages and mental health promotion: what's the connection?

A child's or young person's developmental level can be conceptualised as a 'snapshot at one point in time of the accumulation of predictable-age-related changes that occur in an individual's biological, cognitive, emotional, and social functioning' (Feldman 2001, in Barrett & Ollendick 2004 p. 28). Table 10.1 sets out an overview of developmental stages/tasks for children and young people.

A developmentally oriented treatment and/or management plan needs to take into account the critical developmental tasks and milestones pertinent to a particular child's or adolescent's health problem—for example, self-control and emotion regulation in early childhood or the development of behavioural autonomy and strong peer ties in adolescence (Barrett & Ollendick 2004). Table 10.1 is a conceptual guide only, as in reality the course of developmental changes varies across individuals. Further, some behaviours that are developmentally normative at younger ages (e.g. temper tantrums) are developmentally atypical at later ages. We also know that two young people with similar mental health problems/issues may have developed such problems along very different pathways. The practical application of developmental conceptual models for children and young people is addressed below.

In relation to working therapeutically with children, young people and their families or carers, we know that:

» Positive resolution of developmental tasks moves the adolescent towards adulthood. Assisting the child and adolescent to achieve ego competency skills (Strayhorn 1989, in Stuart & Laraia 1998) and developmental tasks at different stages is the role of significant adults in their lives (e.g. parents, relatives (including grandparents), teachers or foster carers). Parents and primary caregivers can often struggle with understanding the reasonable expectations for a child and adolescent of a particular age. Sometimes, a counsellor or therapist helps the adult carer to fulfil their roles through developing a better understanding of developmental milestones, tasks and expectations. This was certainly the case when working with 13-year-old Chelsea and her mother Vicki. Vicki needed help to understand normative developmental behaviour, not only as it related to Chelsea but also to Chelsea's siblings. Vicki became a more effective parent through being able to distinguish more clearly the different developmental needs of her children (e.g. allowing older children to have a later bedtime or to have a greater say in decision making) and this impacted positively on Chelsea's welfare and emotional wellbeing. See Box 10.3 for a summary of the nine ego competency skills.

» Normal growth and development in children requires a nurturing, supportive environment. Where possible, as you will read in the case with Chelsea and her mum Vicki, it is important to work closely with the parent(s) or primary caregiver(s) towards achieving such an environment; otherwise, individual work done with a young person can be undermined or neutralised. The focus is often on giving praise, setting limits, following logical consequences for inappropriate behaviour and reinforcing desirable behaviours.

Table 10.1 Child and adolescent developmental stages and tasks

Psychosocial development	Cognitive development	Moral development
Preschool		
Starts process of separation and becomes more aware of identity Emerging as social being and able to play alongside other children (parallel play) and with other children (reciprocal play) Identifies with parents of same sex and will copy that parent's behaviour and internalises the attitudes of that parent Has an active imagination and is able to fantasise in play, often using objects in a symbolic manner Will repress unwanted thoughts, experiences and impulses from awareness Can experience a range of emotions, including jealousy, curiosity, joy, grief, affection, anger and fear Developing sense of initiative and dealing with accompanying feelings of guilt Critical period for self-concept development and inner self will be evaluated by what is learned from what others tell them Sees parents as all knowing and all powerful Internalises their family's way of doing and seeing things and this is used to judge their external environment	Learning to use language and represent objects by images and words Egocentric thinking: finds it difficult to accept the viewpoints of others	Recognises good and bad behaviour Understands that they have done something wrong if punished and that if not punished behaviour must be okay
Primary school		
Psychosocial development	**Cognitive development**	**Moral development**
Directs energy towards personal accomplishments, being creative and learning Can tell the difference between fantasy and reality Learning to monitor certain skills with growing confidence Learning to associate performance with rewards and acknowledgment from significant others (e.g. parents/teachers)	Thinking is still egocentric Increasing ability to classify objects and think logically about objects and events	Behaves well if they perceive there is some personal reward (including approval) to be gained Sees good behaviour as that which helps or pleases others

cont.

Table 10.1 Child and adolescent developmental stages and tasks—*cont.*

Psychosocial development	Cognitive development	Moral development
Primary school—*cont.*		
Needs approval from others to confirm self-worth Mastering social and mental skills in school environment Interested in making things and using toy equipment to act out themes that are dominant in their lives Compare themselves socially to peers and are increasingly influenced by them. Learning what they are good at and not so good at Perceptions of friendship developing Able to acknowledge negative and positive aspects of themselves, but often attribute the cause of negative achievements to external sources. With growing ability to be self-critical, may internalise their problems by blaming themselves		Pays little attention to own needs Believes that behaving appropriately is one's duty and that right behaviour is synonymous with obeying rules
Adolescence		
Psychosocial development	**Cognitive development**	**Moral development**
Experiencing great transitional, personal and physical change towards adulthood Developing a more coherent sense of self and emotional independence Absorbed with their own inner world and emotional connectedness Deep emerging concerns about personal appearance, body image, sexuality and the future Often feels helpless, hopeless, sensitive, misunderstood and ignored in their pursuit for independence Can fluctuate between states of extreme happiness and sadness	Able to think logically about abstract propositions and test hypotheses systematically Becomes increasingly concerned with hypothetical propositions, ideological problems and the future	Understands the morality of social contract and accepts laws that protect the rights and welfare of others Avoids violation of rights Internalises moral principles and will voluntarily act in an ethical manner

Note: This table has its foundations in the seminal work of Kohlberg (1963), Piaget (1952) and Erikson (1963, 1968). Their research work addresses the moral, cognitive and psychosocial development of children and adolescents respectively. Kohlberg's levels/stages of moral development are not necessarily linked to particular developmental stages, because certain individuals progress to higher levels of moral development than others.

Source: Adapted from Bigner (1994) and Lewis and Volkmar (1990), cited in Meadows and Singh (2001).

» The young person's search for a unique, new stable identity is very challenging, as the young person is also experiencing dramatic body changes. The search will often require the young person to remaster earlier stages of development (e.g. developing trust in self and others) (Meadows & Singh 2001). Many parents struggle with understanding their adolescent child's simultaneous needs for both dependence and increasing need for independence. The adolescent requires guidelines within which to express growing independence with safety (Meadows & Singh 2001).

» Understanding normal developmental tasks and stages helps the nurse therapist, counsellor or youth worker to identify any marked alterations or deviations in the developmental trajectory for that particular young person. The nurse can pass this understanding on to the parent(s) or caregiver. A child or young person with a mental health illness will often have delayed physical and emotional development.

» Some children and young people find themselves in the situation of being the carer for their parent(s) (e.g. when the parent or caregiver has a long-term physical or mental illness or where there are severe substance abuse problems). Such children who may have been exposed to abuse or violence can experience a role reversal with their parent(s) and develop a pseudomaturity (Stuart & Laraia 1998). The child or young person may appear responsible beyond their years and may be overcompliant with adults. Although seemingly well adapted, this behaviour is developmentally inappropriate and should not be reinforced. The child in this situation needs to be encouraged to choose age-appropriate interests and play activities, and the parent or caregiver needs help to take on appropriate adult responsibilities.

Box 10.3 Ego competency skills

Strayhorn (1989) identified the following nine skills that all children need to become competent adults:

1. establishing closeness and trusting relationships
2. handling separation and independent decision making
3. negotiating joint decisions and interpersonal conflict
4. dealing with frustration and unfavourable events
5. celebrating good feelings and experiencing pleasure
6. working for delayed gratification
7. relaxing and playing
8. cognitive processing through words, symbols and images, and
9. establishing an adaptive sense of direction and purpose.

A focus on ego competency skills is an effective and culturally sensitive way of planning and implementing nursing interventions for young people, regardless of the mental health problem or setting.

Source: Strayhorn (1989), in GW Stuart and MT Laraia 1998 *Principles and practice of psychiatric nursing*, 6th edn. Mosby, St Louis, p. 731.

Vulnerability and resilience

You will recall Chelsea's story from the beginning of the chapter. In order to better understand her situation and needs, it is important to consider the risk and protective factors that contribute to the psychosocial health and wellbeing of children and young people and which interact with developmental tasks. Strong family, school and social supports, productive peer activities, a community that understands and expects changeability and flux, and a young person armed with optimism, hope, resilience and inner strength are all needed. These are all protective factors identified as being effective in preventing the onset of illness and maintaining health and wellbeing. Table 10.2 sets out the risk and protective factors for young people's psychosocial health. (See also Table 1.1 in Ch 1 for a summary of early childhood risk and protective factors.)

Table 10.2 Risk and protective factors influencing the development of psychopatholgy in children and youth

Risk factors	Protective factors
Poor physical health	Physical wellbeing, good nutrition, sleep and exercise
Low self-esteem	Secure, appropriate and safe accommodation
Insecure, inappropriate or unsafe accommodation	Physical and emotional security
Exposure to physical and emotional violence	No harmful alcohol, tobacco and other drug use
Harmful alcohol, tobacco and other drug use	Positive school climate and achievement
Feeling disconnected from family, school and community	Supportive caring parent(s)
Lack of meaningful daily activities	Problem-solving skills
Lack of purpose and meaning in life	Optimism
Lack of control over one's life	Prosocial peers
Financial hardship	Involvement with significant other person
Exposure to environmental stressors (e.g. school bullying)	Availability of opportunities at critical turning points or major life transitions
Poor social skills	Meaningful daily activities
Parental mental illness	Sense of purpose and meaning in life
Learning difficulties	Sense of control and efficacy
Family divorce/separation	Financial security
Ineffective use of medication	Lack of exposure to environmental stressors
	Good coping skills
	Effective use of medication (when required)

Source: Adapted from K Bogenschneider 1996 An ecological risk/protective theory for building prevention programs, policies, and community capacity to support youth. *Family Relations* 45:127–38.

You will note from Table 10.2 that risk and protective factors can be biological, psychological, social or environmental. They can be individual, school related, and/or community and cultural factors. Risk factors are variables that increase the likelihood that disorder will develop and exacerbate the burden of existing disorder (Barrett & Ollendick 2004). Not all children exposed to risk factors go on to develop a mental health disorder (Raphael 2002).

We turn now to Chelsea's story from a clinical point of view, sometimes called a case study. As we explore the treatment and management of Chelsea and her family, it is hoped you will develop a heightened awareness of the inextricable link between treatment and mental health promotion, and an awareness that any uncaring prescriptive implementation of even research-based interventions will not result in the promotion of mental health.

Case study: Chelsea and her family

Chelsea, aged 13, lives with her divorced mother and two siblings—Jessica (aged 8) and Mathew (aged 14), both of whom have physical and developmental problems. Chelsea's father, Brian, lives overseas and separated from the family following domestic violence when Chelsea was aged 7. This violence was witnessed by both Chelsea and Mathew. The contact that the children now have with their father is sporadic telephone contact and is initiated by their mother, Vicki, who feels that the children deserve to maintain some relationship. The family's living situation has been unsettled, since they have had to move three times and so the children have had to leave friends and begin again at new schools.

Chelsea first came to the community mental health clinic when she was 11 years old. At this time her mother was concerned that she had depression. She had always been an unhappy child, but lately she had suicidal ideas and also had behaviours that were difficult to manage. Chelsea also seemed angry, expressing hatred for her family and school. She repeatedly told her mother that she wanted to die and wrote notes both at home and at school saying she wished she was dead. Additionally, it was reported that, at school, Chelsea was the victim of bullying from an older girl. The school teacher was concerned about Chelsea's achievement and development. She always seemed to look unhappy and had missed a lot of days due to physical illnesses such as colds and middle ear infections.

Vicki appeared to lack confidence in her parenting role. She did not feel effective in the ways she managed each child's oppositional behaviour. She also failed to consistently set limits for the children and did not always follow through with logical consequences for unreasonable behaviour. Nor did she notice desirable behaviour and reinforce / reward it. Vicki also tended to take it personally when her children acted badly. She had a habit of blaming the children if she had a bad week or if things were stressful or tense at home. Generally, there were many conflicts at home—between siblings, and between the mother and children. There were also financial pressures. At the time, Vicki was not seeing her own counsellor, despite being diagnosed with depression, and she had few friends. There was no immediate family support because all the other relatives live in a different state.

Planning a comprehensive model of care

This is a true story. Indeed, it is a common one that faces mental health clinicians working with young people. Chelsea has depression, which is the most frequently reported mental health problem in young people, and indeed the general population. All over the world, society is facing what amounts to an epidemic of depression. It is now the second leading cause of death and disease, after heart disease (Murray & Lopez 1997, Lopez et al. 2006). Early onset depression has been linked to a variety of negative outcomes in childhood and in later adolescence, including increased risk of suicide attempts, not completing school, teenage pregnancy and mood disturbance into adulthood (Seligman & Ollendick 1998).

This story also reveals that mental health issues are just as much social and environmental, as they can be biological and individual. They involve interplay between factors that affect the wellbeing of the young person, their family, peers and social networks. For Chelsea and her family, what happens now and in the future, as well as reflecting on what happened in the past, is vital for their long-term mental health and adaptation. In mental health care, the aim is not simply to relieve present symptoms, such as Chelsea's suicidal ideas, or to resolve deficiencies, such as Vicki's parenting style. These are likely to be short-term solutions and problems are likely to re-emerge. A longer term, more effective and holistic approach is to use a model of care that values prevention of mental disorder and dysfunction, taking early intervention on any bio-psychosocial issues, and active promotion of recovery and adaptation.

Helping Chelsea, as well as other young people feeling depressed and overwhelmed, requires much more than a treatment model. Reflecting on the principles of mental health promotion previously discussed, the approach needs to have an environmental as well as individual focus that reaches across the whole spectrum of interventions. In particular, three strategies are needed:

1. *prevention strategies* that target risk and protective factors amenable to intervention and which are able to reduce the onset of new cases of depression
2. *treatment and management strategies* that better respond to and lessen the burden on young people currently suffering depression, and
3. *recovery strategies* that assist individuals and facilitate community participation, to ensure control over health-related behaviours.

Prevention strategies

Even though direct causes of most mental disorders remain unknown, nurses can be active in modifying and reducing risks and enhancing protective influences across every stage of the lifespan (for an overview of these lifespan issues, see Raphael 2002). In order to prevent the actual onset of disorders such as depression, *universal prevention strategies* are recommended. These are strategies that raise the whole society's awareness of ways to promote mental health or to build resilience and prevent problems.

One example is 'Beyond Blue', an Australian national depression initiative. One of its projects provides mental health education so that children, parents and school personnel have raised awareness of issues and information to identify problems and seek help for themselves (Burns & Field 2002). In New Zealand, programs like 'Strengthening Families' and 'Family Start' (www.mhc.govt.nz) are working to build family effectiveness so that children are more likely to be raised in nurturing environments, thus strengthening their resistance to stressors. Media awareness campaigns that encourage people to enjoy life and find ways to reduce stress are other examples of universal interventions.

Prevention also involves targeting specific interventions towards *selected* groups known to be at-risk. For example, children of parents with affective illness, especially depression, compared to children of non-depressed parents, are at greater risk of developing anxiety disorders, major depression and substance dependence (Weissman et al. 2006). Depressed parents are often emotionally unavailable to their children. In turn, as found in the Tasmanian Children's Project (Handley et al. 2001), these children can become 'parentified' as they take on the mantle of adult responsibilities normally borne by the parent. Such children are at risk of developing a range of mental disorders and comprise a vulnerable group. They are also at risk of inconsistent parenting if their parents are themselves unstable and adhering sporadically to treatment. Such children benefit from selected prevention strategies—those that work with them early on in their illness, helping them to maintain and develop inner strengths, and treat problems early.

A well-researched Australian *selective intervention* program for young people with anxiety is the FRIENDS program (Barrett et al. 2000a, 2000b, 2000c) designed for children and young people aged between 7 and 11 years and between 12 and 16 years. FRIENDS is an acronym for **F**eelings; **R**elax and feel good; **I**nner helpful thoughts; **E**xplore plans; **N**ice work, reward yourself; **D**on't forget to practice; **S**tay calm. This program can be implemented by all those working with youth, following participation in an accredited training workshop (Barrett & Ollendick 2004). Using a combination of cognitive, family and interpersonal therapies, the aim is for children to recognise links between thoughts and feelings, manage stress and develop coping strategies. For Chelsea, the aim might be to help her deal with fallouts with friends and siblings, cope with changing school, going on a camp and going to hospital.

Indicated strategies are those that target prevention towards high-risk groups, such as those who show early signs of illness, a high number of risk factors for a given illness, or biological markers known to predispose them to mental disorder. In Australia, the Early Psychosis Prevention and Intervention Centre (EPPIC) early intervention program for first case psychosis is a good example. In this program, nurses and others actively follow up a client who may have been recently discharged, and offer them assistance in treatment adherence, facilitated peer-support groups, leisure skills, supported employment and carer involvement. Such measures are known to reduce severity, disability, relapse and costs associated with schizophrenia-type disorders (Paterson et al. 2001).

Treatment strategies

The specific interventions that make up mental health treatment involve a whole range of health promoting practices, including assessment and diagnosis, application of evidence-based interventions, holistic care, collaboration and partnership, and family-sensitive service delivery. In reality, 'treatment' cannot be separated from any of these elements. Next, each of these different aspects will be discussed in relation to Chelsea's situation.

During assessment and on an ongoing basis, a mental status examination is completed. We would recommend that any nurse working with young people develop the requisite skills to complete a basic mental health status examination, even if as a result you decide to refer on to a mental health professional. An important aspect of mental health promotion is recognising personal and professional limitations with regard to treating young people who are demonstrating signs of dysfunction.

Much of the data for such an assessment will emerge spontaneously (appearance, mood/affect and thought processes), while other data will be gathered via structured questioning and activities (Meadows & Singh 2001). Identifying the young person's positive attributes is central to taking a mental health promotion stance towards mental health assessment. For example, can the young person problem-solve? What are their strengths and interests? How do they deal with stress? How well do they understand the problem that brought them to you? What do they think caused the problem? How upset are they about the problem? What are their views about the possible solutions?

Although questions like these guided the assessment of Chelsea, the process is of course ongoing, and preliminary clinical impressions may shift with time. In our experience, assessment tools are most useful in helping clinicians explore and interpret the client's behaviour and needs. When they are used rigidly or restrictively, when they close down communication between client and clinician, then they function as barriers to the therapeutic relationship. Thus, it is important to use questions carefully, and use tools when and only when they assist in helping you get to know the person more clearly and deeply.

It emerged over time, for example, that Chelsea had depression as well as anxiety. Anxiety in childhood may play a causal role in the development of depression in young people (Seligman & Ollendick 1998). Chelsea also experienced many complicating risk factors, including financial hardship, school bullying, maternal depression and a pessimistic temperament. At the same time, though, certain protective factors also emerged at initial assessment and in ongoing sessions with Chelsea and her mother. Chelsea was achieving well in most subjects at school, she did have friends, she was a very bright and questioning child, she had a supportive mother even though her mother was struggling with her own depression and could be overly critical of Chelsea, she had a good relationship with one of her teachers at school, and she was involved in dancing and netball activities, which she liked.

Evidenced-based interventions

The *National action plan for promotion, prevention and early intervention for mental health* (National Mental Health Strategy 2000) outlines the evidence base for promoting mental health and reducing mental health problems and disorders for children aged 5–11 years and young people aged 12–17 years and their parents. In Australia, interventions in both the home and school settings that have been effective in preventing mental health problems in these age groups are identified. This document also poses some critical research questions that are still as relevant in 2007 as they were in 2000. For example:

- Which interventions enhance resilience in children?
- What screening tools validly and reliably identify the early signs and symptoms of emerging mental health problems in children?
- How can an at-risk mental state be reliably identified in young people?
- What prevention and early intervention programs are effective for eating disorders and substance misuse in young people?
- What are the most effective strategies for young people no longer at school?
- What are the effects and side-effects of using medication for early intervention with young people, particularly for psychosis and depression?

It is important to point out that some treatments for young people are more effective than others and different treatment strategies can be effective with one young person and not another. Well-established efficacious treatments for children and young people include behavioural parent training for ADHD (attention deficit hyperactivity disorder) and ODD (oppositional defiant disorder) and graduated exposure for phobias (Barrett & Ollendick 2004). Cognitive behavioural therapy is described as probably efficacious for anxiety, depression and autism. More work needs to be done to establish efficaciousness of these and other interventions such as psychodynamic psychotherapies or family systems therapies (Ollendick & King 2000).

Treatment strategies for adolescents often include medication, supportive counselling, and/or a range of psychodynamic therapies, including symbolic, expressive strategies to help the young person talk about difficult issues in ways that are less direct and more metaphorical. Sandplay, art, role-play, clay therapy and dreamwork are examples. Therapeutic tools that are not dependent on high levels of verbal articulation are better suited to meeting the challenges posed by resistant or defensive clients or those less articulate. In addition, behavioural and cognitive behavioural strategies are useful for encouraging self-belief and self-control, to challenge self-destructive beliefs, manage anger, teach assertion, and encourage the setting of life goals. Psycho-educational approaches are also useful in explaining some of the psychosocial issues about fluctuating hormones and moods and relationships.

For more information, readers are encouraged to access Geldard and Geldard (1999) who provide a detailed and practice-based exploration of a wide range of counselling and therapy strategies for emotionally disturbed children and adolescents.

The treatment plan for Chelsea included the use of medication to help with her anxiety and depression, combined with a cognitive-behavioural and psycho-educational approach. Box 10.4 provides a summary of common interventions for young people, including those used with Chelsea.

Psycho-educational strategies involved both Chelsea and her mum, Vicki, and addressed the topics of anxiety and depression, as well as the issues of stigma related to mental illness. It took some time for Vicki to acknowledge that she was suffering from depression. Her acceptance of this diagnosis and consequent treatment played an important part in Chelsea's recovery. In order to promote improved mental health for Chelsea, these approaches needed to be specifically tailored to her needs, taking into account on a session-by-session basis her energy levels, motivation, interests and connectedness with the therapist.

Holism

In mental health care, treatment approaches value taking into account the uniqueness of each person. In nursing you would be familiar with the biopsychosocial framework. Another useful assessment framework guiding holistic assessment and treatment for young people is the HEADSS Psychosocial Assessment (see Table 10.3). According to the National Divisions Youth Alliance (2004), this framework is part of the Adolescent Health Check template developed by the Australian General Practice Network.

In applying holism to the care and management of Chelsea and her family, it was important to consider the home situation. For example, Chelsea shared a room

Box 10.4 Commonly used interventions with children and adolescents

Behaviour therapy
Behaviour modification programs are designed to motivate and reward age-appropriate behaviours by using, for example, points or privileges. Most parent training programs are based on behavioural principles.

Cognitive-behavioural therapy (CBT)
The goal of CBT is to modify maladaptive or unhelpful ways of thinking and behaving with more positive ways of thinking and behaving. Clients may be asked to record their thoughts and become more aware of how their thinking style affects their feeling and behaviour. Other strategies include cognitive rehearsal, social skills and assertiveness training, and relaxation techniques.

Play therapy
Play therapy usually refers to one-to-one sessions with a child in a playroom. Most playrooms are equipped with art supplies, clay or play dough, dolls and puppets. Through play, a child learns to master impulses and adapt to the environment.

Psychoeducational therapy
This is a strategy of teaching clients and their families about disorders, treatments, coping techniques and resources. It helps empower clients and families by having them become more involved and prepares them to participate in their own care once they have the necessary knowledge.

Expressive therapy
Expressive therapies include innovative artistic therapies such as art, clay, dance, movement, music and drama, which can contribute significantly to the therapeutic process, especially for the non-articulate, defensive or resistive client.

Source: E Varcarolis, V Carson and E Shoemaker 2006 *Foundations of psychiatric mental health nursing: a clinical approach.* Elsevier, St Louis.

with her younger sister and as Chelsea grew older this had become problematic. Yet, realistically, her mum could simply not afford a bigger house. This became something the whole team needed to think creatively about. In addition, Chelsea's education, eating and exercise were considered. It emerged that she was being bullied by an older girl at school. This was causing major distress for Chelsea. It was eroding her self-confidence and impacting on her learning capabilities and her grades at school. The impact of the bullying was so great that a decision by her mother to change schools was supported by her therapist. As time has gone on, the change in schools enhanced Chelsea's life considerably and has become a key protective factor for her ongoing wellbeing.

Chelsea had a good appetite and areas like sleep were not severely disrupted, but she did benefit from becoming more aware of the importance of healthy food and exercise as a way of increasing her physical health and enhancing her mood and wellbeing. Chelsea's involvement in out-of-school activities and friendships

Table 10.3 HEADSS framework for adolescents

H: Home—consider living arrangements, relationships, childhood events, abuse, cultural identity, recent life events, community supports

E: Education, Employment, Eating and Exercise—consider school/work retention, bullying, study/career progress and goals, nutrition, eating patterns, weight gain/loss, energy, fitness/exercise

A: Activities, Hobbies and Peer Relationships—consider hobbies, peer groups, activities, venues, lifestyle factors, risk-taking, injury avoidance

D: Drug Use—consider cigarette smoking, substance use/abuse, quantity, frequency, tolerance, withdrawal, prescription drugs, treatment adherence, preparedness for change

S: Sexual Activity and Sexuality—consider sexual activity, age of onset, safe sex practices, same sex attraction, pap smear date/sexually transmitted infections screening, sexual abuse, pregnancy/children

S: Suicide, Depression and Risk—consider anxiety, depression, self-harm, reaction to stress, tension and release strategies, mental state examination, risk assessment: plan of suicide, current or past, risk to others

Mental state examination

Perceptions (hallucinations, illusions)
Orientation (time, place, person)
Affect (apparent feeling state: relaxed, sad, blunted, flat)
Thoughts (looseness, logic, absence, content, delusions, obsessions, fears)
Mood (internal emotion: depressed, elated)
Judgment (ability to make rational decision)
Speech (rate, stutters and volume)
Insight (knowledge of condition)
General appearance (dishevelled, odd)
Memory (short, long, recall)
Intelligence

Source: Adapted from J Goldenring & E Cohen 1988 Getting into adolescents' heads. *Contemporary Pediatrics* July:75–80.

was also encouraged. Her mother was encouraged to allow Chelsea to go on a holiday to visit relatives. This provided fun, safe independence, as well as much needed respite. Drug use and sexual activity were not an issue with Chelsea, though ongoing assessment in relation to suicidal ideation, depression and safety were integral to the ongoing management of Chelsea. Consider the critical questions and reflections in Box10.5 to further explore holism.

Box 10.5 Critical questions and reflections: exploring holism

1. To what extent do the health systems with which you are familiar operate in this 'whole of society' approach to health promotion and illness prevention?
2. What practices can community-based nurses begin to take up based on the range of interventions discussed?

Partnership and collaboration

Effective treatment and management of emotional distress in young people, within the context of mental health promotion and recovery, will more often than not involve you as a nurse counsellor or therapist collaborating with, and working in partnership with, a number of stakeholders, including parents, teachers, general practitioners, paediatricians, guidance counsellors and child and family services. The inclusion of parents and family members in the treatment programs for young people with depression is currently the subject of empirical research measuring responses to treatment of young people who have shown poor response rates to even the best treatments. This seems sensible given that families of depressed children often exhibit family dysfunction and may have parents who have their own psychopathology. Early findings indicate that parental psychopathology is a significant moderator of treatment efficacy (Brent & Kolko 1998).

In Chelsea's case, where her mother also has depression, it is imperative to work in a family-sensitive manner, ever mindful of the shame, secrecy and stigma associated with parental mental illness and how this impacts on the children. Strategies need to be non-blaming, using understanding, respect, openness and education. Where a child is being placed at risk through any form of abuse related to the parent's mental illness or reduced coping capacities, it is still possible to work in positive and solution-focused ways.

It was possible, for example, to arrange short-term intensive family support to provide respite and reinforce effective parenting strategies. The challenge was to assist Vicki to see this intervention as a positive support and not a blaming response to the sometimes ineffective ways she managed the challenges she faced as a single parent struggling with a mental illness herself. Chelsea became happier, less angry and more optimistic as Vicki became more confident in her role as parent and sought help for her depression.

Continuing care or recovery strategies

It is possible for all people to *recover* from mental health problems, even if some symptoms might recur now and then. Recovery is an important and overarching principle that underpins rehabilitation work and continuing care. It really means the development of new meaning and purpose in one's life as one grows beyond (and perhaps despite) the effects of mental illness. It means maximising wellbeing, within the constraints that might be imposed by symptoms of mental illness.

However, some people may experience ongoing mental health problems, or if they do not adhere to treatments they are at risk of relapse. In these cases, continuing care that provides optimism and active ongoing skill development is known to be effective.

Raising the public's awareness of the rights and needs of people with mental health problems is an important strategy in this phase. This strategy has potential to reduce the stigma of mental disorders. Stigma can lead to discrimination, alienation, loneliness and rejection. So any anti-stigma practices have the effect of optimising people's mental health by creating environments that support wellbeing. In addition, activities that support people in continuing care are all ways to facilitate recovery.

Awareness programs are important and an example is the Headroom website (www.headroom.net.au), which has mental health resources developed by young people for young people. Chelsea and Vicki were helped to become more aware of their symptoms of depression and anxiety, the early warning signs and their associated risk and protective factors. Alternatives to hospital programs are also useful and an example is Stepping Stones (see www.steppingstoneclubhouse.org.au), which provides a recovery program in a non-institutional setting where young adults with a mental disorder provide support to each other as they work to rebuild their confidence, self-esteem, social and vocational skills.

Chelsea was encouraged to explore a range of cognitive behavioural strategies to deal with her negative emotions and thinking, including thought records, keeping a diary, and pleasant events schedules. She was also encouraged to see events like sleepovers, swimming, dancing and camps as important supports for her overall wellbeing. Timely medical intervention to assist with Chelsea's recurring ear infections contributed to her overall wellbeing, including a decrease in her depression and sense of hopelessness about life.

Conclusion

It is not always easy working with children and young people who have mental health issues, but it is important to remember that it also is not easy growing up. Perhaps it is useful to remember that we were all young once, and understanding and working with children and particularly young people requires genuine empathy. The art of being a good clinician, effective in promoting mental health and wellbeing, is to be knowledgeable, concernful, nurturing and ready to provide support. As Burgess (2006) said:

> 'Growing things are so interesting. It should be a pleasure to review a time when we were changing so much, growing, learning so much. We have a lot to learn from teenagers about how to keep on our toes, about how to be lazy, about how to be playful, and most of all, how to just grow up.'

Practice tips

- » Growing up is a time of rapid change and adaptation. Physical, hormonal, role, relationship and thinking changes can fluctuate wildly, creating tension and stress.
- » Young people may be vulnerable to feelings of anxiety and depression and may need assistance from empathic, supportive, skilled clinicians who understand this life transition.
- » Risk and protective factors shape the balance of vulnerabilities and strengths for children and young people, potentially influencing their psychosocial health.
- » The spectrum of interventions in mental health is a useful model to guide a whole-of-society approach to mental health promotion and illness prevention.
- » Mental health promotion strategies for young people are integral to effective treatment and management and include collaborative and family-sensitive practices.

» Opportunities for practice development include enhancing integrated care that follows clients through from prevention, to treatment, to continuing care or support in their recovery; and in developing solution-oriented models of care that harness clients' strengths, involve young people in the service that they are using, and convey hope and optimism for change.

Useful resources

Australia

Australian Network for Promotion, Prevention and Early Intervention for Mental Health (Auseinet): www.auseinet.com.au.

Beyond Blue, the national depression initiative devoted to increasing awareness and understanding of depression in the community: www.beyondblue.org.au/.

COPMI (Children of Parents with a Mental Illness), a comprehensive directory of resources targeted to the needs of young children 0–6 years, primary children 7–12 years, young people 13–18 years, parents, teachers, community workers and child protection/justice and workforce educators: www.copmi.net.au.

Headroom (cubbyhouse), which helps younger kids to understand and deal with things like friendship, bullying and stress: www.headroom.net.au. The 'lounge' link is for adolescents and has been written by young people for young people.

'It's all right', a SANE website for young people with family or friends affected by mental illness: www.itsallright.org.

Kids Help Line, a free, confidential and anonymous 24-hour telephone and online counselling service to children and adolescents in Australia aged 5–18 years: www.kidshelp.com.au.

Mindmatters, a national project that uses universal prevention strategies to raise awareness of mental health and lifestyle issues in school children: www.mindmatters.org.au.

National mental health plan and strategy: www.health.gov.au.

New South Wales Centre for the Advancement of Adolescent Health: www.caah.chw.edu.au/resources/.

Reachout, a national initiative that uses the internet to reach out to all young people, giving information and referrals in a format that appeals to young people: www.reachout.com.au.

Europe and the United Kingdom

European mental health implementation project: http://mentalhealth.epha.org/.

National Institute for Mental Health in England: http://nimhe.csip.org.uk/home.

National Program for Improving Mental Health and Wellbeing in Scotland: www.wellscotland.com.

New Zealand

Mental Health Foundation of New Zealand, a national organisation that provides information and resources, and disseminates research activities: http://mentalhealth.org.nz.

MindNet.org.NZ, an online resource on mental health promotion and prevention activities: www.mindnet.org.nz/.

References

Aspinwall L, Staudinger U (eds) 2003 *A psychology of human strengths: fundamental questions and future directions for a positive psychology*. American Psychological Association, Washington DC.

Barrett P, Lowry-Webster H, Turner C 2000a *Friends for children group leader manual*. Australian Academic Press, Brisbane.

Barrett P, Lowry-Webster H, Turner C 2000b *Friends for children participants workbook*. Australian Academic Press, Brisbane.

Barrett P, Lowry-Webster H, Turner C 2000c *Friends for youth group participants manual*. Australian Academic Press, Brisbane.

Barrett P, Ollendick T (eds) 2004 *Handbook of interventions that work with children and adolescents: prevention and treatment*. Johns Wiley & Sons, West Sussex.

Bogenschneider K 1996 An ecological risk/protective theory for building prevention programs, policies, and community capacity to support youth. *Family Relations* 45:127–38.

Bowles N, Mackintosh C, Torn A 2001 Nurses' communication skills: an evaluation of the impact of solution-focused communication training. *Journal of Advanced Nursing* 36:347–54.

Brent D, Kolko D 1998 Psychotherapy: definitions, mechanisms of action, and relationship to etiological models. *Journal of Abnormal Child Psychology* 26(1):17–26.

Burgess M 2006 Then, thank god we grew up. *The Guardian*, 27 May. Available at www.guardian.co.uk/family/story/0,,17830351,00.html. Accessed 27 May 2006.

Burns J, Field K 2002 Beyond Blue: targeting depression in young people. *Youth Studies Australia* 21:43–51.

Carradice A, Round D 2004 Practice development. The reality of practice development for nurses working in an inpatient service for people with severe and enduring mental health problems. *Journal of Psychiatric and Mental Health Nursing* 11:731–7.

Erikson E 1963 *Childhood and society*, 2nd edn. WW Norton, New York.

Erikson E 1968 *Identity, youth and crises*. WW Norton, New York.

Geldard K, Geldard D 1999 *Counselling adolescents*. Sage, London.

Goldenring J, Cohen E 1988 Getting into adolescents' heads. *Contemporary Pediatrics* July:75–80.

Handley C, Farrell G, Josephs A et al. 2001 The Tasmanian children project: the needs of children with a parent/carer with a mental illness. *Australian and New Zealand Journal of Mental Health Nursing* 10:221–8.

Happell B, Manias E, Pinikahana J 2002 The role of the inpatient mental health nurse in facilitating adherence to medication regimes. *International Journal of Mental Health Nursing* 11:251–9.

Kohlberg L 1963 The development of children's orientations toward moral order: sequence in the development of moral thought. *Vita Humana* 6(11):33–173.

Lopez A, Mathers C, Ezzati M et al. (eds) 2006 *Global burden of disease and risk factors*. World Bank, Washington DC.

Meadows G, Singh B (eds) 2001 *Mental health in Australia: collaborative community practice*. Oxford University Press, Melbourne.

Mental Health Commission 1998 *Blueprint for mental health services in New Zealand: how things need to be*. Mental Health Commission, Wellington.

Mindframe n.d. *Mental illness facts and figures*. Available at www.mindframe-media.info/mi/stats_more.php. Accessed 14 October 2006.

Mrazek P, Haggerty R (eds) 1994 *Reducing risks for mental disorders: frontiers for intervention research*. National Academy Press, Washington DC.

Murray C, Lopez A 1997 Global mortality, disability and the contribution of risk factors: global burden of disease study. *The Lancet* 349(9063):1436–42.

National Divisions Youth Alliance 2004 *HEADSS psychosocial assessment*. Available at http://ndya.adgp.com.au/site/index.cfm?display=2456. Accessed 8 January 2006.

National Mental Health Strategy 2000 *National action plan for promotion, prevention and early intervention for mental health 2000*. Department of Health and Ageing, Canberra.

Ollendick T, King N 2000 Empirically supported treatments for children and adolescents. In PC Kendall (ed.), *Child and adolescent therapy: cognitive behavioural procedures*, 2nd edn. Guilford Publications, New York, pp. 386–425.

Paterson K, Jones J, Dagg B et al. 2001 Getting in early: a framework for early intervention and prevention in mental health for young people in New South Wales. *NSW Public Health Bulletin* 12:137.

Piaget J 1952 *The origins of intelligence in children*. Translated by Margaret Cook, International Universities Press, New York.

Raphael B 2002 Children, young people and families: a population health approach to mental health. *Youth Studies Australia* 21:12–16.

Resnick M, Bearman P, Blum R et al. 1997 Protecting adolescents from harm: findings from the national longitudinal study on adolescent health. *Journal of the American Medical Association* 278:823–32.

SANE Australia 2004 *Dare to care! SANE mental health report*. Sane Australia, Melbourne. Available at www.sane.org. Accessed 14 May 2005.

Sawyer M, Arney F, Baghurst P et al. 2000 *The mental health of young people in Australia*. AGPS, Canberra.

Seligman L, Ollendick T 1998 Comorbidity of anxiety and depression in children and adolescents: an integrative review. *Clinical Child and Family Psychology Review* 1:125–144.

Stacey K, Webb E, Hills S et al. 2002 Relationships and power. *Youth Studies Australia* 21:44–51.

Stuart G, Laraia M 1998 *Principles and practice of psychiatric nursing*, 6th edn. Mosby, St Louis.

Webb L 2002 Deliberate self-harm in adolescence: a systematic review of psychological and psychosocial factors. *Journal of Advanced Nursing* 38:235–44.

Weissman M, Wickramaratne P, Nomura Y et al. 2006 Offspring of depressed parents: 20 years later. *American Journal of Psychiatry* 163:1001–9.

World Health Organization (WHO) 2001 *The world health report 2001—mental health: new understanding, new hope*. WHO, Geneva.

Wright R, Cummings N (eds) 2005 *Destructive trends in mental health: the well-intentioned path to harm*. Routledge, New York.

Chapter 11

Loss and grief

Elizabeth Forster and Judith Murray

Learning outcomes

Reading this chapter will help you to:

- » discuss the concepts of grief and loss
- » describe factors that influence grief responses
- » describe differences between sudden and anticipated loss
- » discuss anticipatory grief
- » discuss parental grief
- » discuss developmental differences in relation to children's understanding of death and their grief responses, and
- » describe supportive ways to interact with parents and siblings in the context of loss.

Introduction

Grieving is a normal human process of healing that involves a person dealing with the variable pain of being separated from someone or something of importance to them, and adjusting to a world in which that valued person or thing is missing. Such adjustment involves an ability to integrate that which was lost into the ongoing life of the person so the lost person or thing is removed from a central role in daily functioning, while its possible ongoing effect on the individual remains recognised and respected. Understanding grief and loss as concepts within the context of caring for children, young people and families is important, as appropriate responses and understanding are required at this extraordinary time.

Setting the scene: a clinical scenario

You are working in a maternity ward where you are caring for 40-year-old Jacqui who has just given birth to a baby girl, Julie, who was stillborn. Jacqui learnt a few days ago during her antenatal appointment that her baby had died in utero when the baby's heartbeat could not be detected. She was then admitted to the labour ward and labour was induced. Jacqui is accompanied by her husband Mark and her step-children Alex, aged 4 years, and John, aged 14 years. Jacqui had been undergoing fertility treatment for 3 years prior to Julie's birth and had suffered numerous miscarriages.

Defining loss, grief and bereavement

A burgeoning theory and research base concerning grief and bereavement has arisen in the past few decades. A useful starting point in coming to understand this literature is to reflect upon definitions of grief, bereavement and loss, as well as the themes and trends in current research.

Although many definitions exist in the literature, for the purposes of this chapter, bereavement involves the loss of someone or something. The term has often been confined to the event of loss through death. However, it is also used to describe not only the event but also the internal and external processes of adaptation of individuals and family members across the many facets of the experience around death. This includes the anticipation of the loss, the loss itself and the experiences of adjustment following this loss (Genevro et al. 2004 p. 498). These dual processes of bereavement that include the internal processes of adaptation to the death itself such as dealing with separation anxiety and finding meaning, as well as the external processes of adaptation or restoration-oriented activities that may involve relationship changes and living arrangement changes, both occur following the loss (Stroebe & Schut 1999).

Raphael (1984) defines grief as the emotional responses to loss: the complex amalgam of painful effects, including sadness, anger, helplessness, guilt and despair. While many commonalities exist, individuals vary in their experience of grief—in its intensity, its duration and its means of expression (Murray 2005a, Genevro et al. 2004). Some people may not experience distress or display grief responses anticipated by others. However, such responses do not necessarily indicate some problem in grieving (Wortman & Silver 2001). In some cases, loss may represent the end of a burden and result in a lesser degree of distress for the person. In other cases, previous life experiences may have led to the person being less fearful of the grief experienced and hence less distressed. In fact, the experience of loss can bring forth positive emotions and changes to the affected person(s) (Calhoun & Tedeschi 2006).

While the term 'bereavement' refers to situations involving death, the more general term of 'loss' refers to situations over which people grieve. Loss has been defined most simply as the experience of being parted from something or someone of value. More formally, Miller and Omarzu (1998) define loss as the experience of being separated from that of value in that loss is 'produced by an event which is perceived to be negative by the individuals involved and results in long-term changes to one's social situations, relationships, or cognitions' (p. 12).

As such, it may not be confined to a single event, but may encompass an ongoing set of events. In being parted from something of value to us, complete dissociation from the lost object may never fully occur and the 'something' over which a person may grieve is defined by the person experiencing the loss, rather than others. Therefore, grief and loss are not confined to loss through the death of a loved one. It includes events that are an inevitable part of life's journey, such as those associated with ageing or moving from primary to secondary school, or the private, less tangible losses that human beings experience such as missing out on a job, being betrayed by a friend or unrequited love. Loss may also include deprivation or neglect such as homelessness, disability or abuse (Murray 2005a).

Current trends in thinking on grief and loss

Most schools of psychological thought have had something to say about grieving, with most proposing explanatory models. There have been contributions from psychodynamic theory (Freud 1917), attachment theory (Bowlby 1961, Kübler-Ross 1969, Parkes 1972, Raphael 1984), social learning theory (Doka 1989, Glick et al. 1974), and personal construct theory (Neimeyer & Mahoney 1995).

Traditional models of grief, such as the phases and stages model proposed by Elisabeth Kübler Ross (1969), have had widespread appeal, as they assist in illuminating the experience of loss. However, these models have limited empirical support, as grieving individuals demonstrate varied responses to loss rather than progressing through distinct stages or sequences of psychological states (Neimeyer 2000). Often these models have been seen as competing for influence in the discussions of grief, when, in reality, each theory has added more to our understanding of this important human experience.

The early theorists provided the basic understandings in describing the process of mourning. In later times, others have added understanding, provided greater clarity, or made corrections when empirical data or new theory contradicted accepted understandings. Some models have combined the theoretical emphases of different schools. For example, the task-based models of mourning (Worden 1991, Rando 1993) were a combination of the psychodynamic concepts of grief work and the phasic models of attachment theories. More recent integrated models such as the Four Components Model (Bonanno & Kaltmann 1999) and the Dual Process Model (Stroebe & Schut 1999) have sought to employ the knowledge of many schools of thought.

Assumptive worlds

Another perspective that offers much to the understanding of grief and loss is that of *assumptive worlds*. Parkes (1975 p. 132) defined the assumptive world as:

> 'The individual's view of reality as he believes it to be, i.e., a strongly held set of assumptions about the world and the self which are confidently maintained and used as a means of recognizing, planning and acting.'

Assumptions are learned and confirmed through the life experiences of each individual. They are learned within the contexts of living within families, community and culture, as well as through individual life experiences. Essentially, assumptions are those understandings of the world that are reinforced over time by certain events and interactions. As such, assumptions can be both positive and negative, and become the filter through which people interpret their world and events that happen in it.

These assumptions provide the individual with the ability to make predictions about the world and so order their behaviour to conform to this world. Such predictability provides a sense of security in living everyday life. Janoff-Bulman (1992) argues that in western civilisations, individuals hold three basic assumptions:

1. the world is benevolent (or malevolent)
2. the world is meaningful (or meaningless), and
3. the self is worthy (or unworthy).

Some life events challenge the security of the world and challenge assumptions. Parkes (1988 p. 55) defined psychosocial transitions as life events:

> '. . . that a) require people to undertake a major revision of their assumptions of the world, b) are lasting in their implications rather than transient, and c) take place over a relatively short period of time so that there is little opportunity for preparation.'

For many people, illness and death are psychosocial transitions. Parkes (1975) argues that there are different responses within the worldview to psychosocial transitions. The former view of the world, or at least some aspects of it, can be abandoned, which may lead to either a satisfactory or a frightening outcome, depending on whether the event seriously threatens the sense of security. But some may refuse to abandon this worldview and hence try to maintain it by trying to force the current world, or parts thereof, to conform to the previous assumptive world. Sometimes, the old assumptive world remains unchanged and exists alongside the new world. The individual then oscillates between the two worlds—for example, when a person maintains hope for health in the face of increasing evidence of a degenerating condition.

Certain types of deaths are more likely to shatter one's assumptive world, including deaths that are sudden or without warning or those that occur because of a deliberate act (Davis et al. 2000), deaths that are untimely, such as the death of a child or the loss of a spouse at a young age. These deaths shatter fundamental assumptions—for example, that children should outlive their parents, and that children should grow into adults and lead long and happy lives.

In response to these losses, the bereaved may embark upon a search for meaning that involves reaching a new understanding—a 'relearning' and 'reinvesting' in the world that has changed because of the loss of the loved one (Wheeler 2001). As well as relearning or reconciling one's world from the past to the present and future in light of their loss, the bereaved person may also need to find renewed purpose and reason in living (Wheeler 2001).

Sudden versus expected loss and anticipatory grief

Death may be expected or unexpected, the characteristics of which differ and can influence the impact on survivors. According to Iserson (2000), characteristics that may differ depending on whether the death is expected or not include the cause of death, the age of the deceased, when and where the death occurs, the involvement and reaction of the survivors, the site of last contact with health professionals, resuscitation, autopsy requirements, and immediate family rituals and requirements.

The family members in the case scenario are coming to terms with the sudden and unexpected loss of their long-awaited baby. In a sudden unexpected death, the family may have only a very short time of preparation or no warning at all. The place of death may be in a public place, at home or at work, or in an emergency department or intensive care unit. Family members may or may not be present at the time of death and may be contacted and gather gradually. The family may have witnessed resuscitation procedures and may need to discuss autopsy requirements soon after their loved one's death. In some cases, coronial requirements may prevent easy and unlimited access to the person who has died or may necessitate the involvement of the police as the investigative arm of the Coroner. All this often occurs when a person is dealing with the reactions of shock that can compromise their ability to assimilate and deal with all that is required of them.

In contrast, when the death of a loved one is expected, it usually occurs following a long chronic or life-threatening illness and may occur at home or in a hospital or aged care facility. The death usually occurs weeks, months or years following the original diagnosis, and family members may have had some time to prepare and are often present at the time of death (Iserson 2000).

The many potential differences between sudden, unexpected and expected loss have the potential to influence the relationship between health professionals and bereaved families and the nature of support provided following loss. Paediatric death introduces additional complexities.

When the death of a child is sudden and unexpected, health professionals have a limited timeframe in which to initiate support and must provide this support to parents/families experiencing overwhelming and intense shock and grief. This may not only limit the amount and type of support health professionals can offer, but also have a negative impact on their perceived ability to provide this support. Following sudden or accidental death, many variables will influence the severity of shock families experience: the child who died as a person, when he or she died, the relationship or degree of attachment between the parents and family and the deceased child, and the coping ability of the parents and family members (Sanders 1986). Sanders (1986) also highlights that the manner in which health professionals impart the news of the death to relatives can have long-lasting and negative effects on their bereavement and leave them feeling guilty or shocked if the news was delivered in an insensitive way.

Perinatal death in itself is also different to some extent from other child death in that the whole event of pregnancy is involved. Perinatal death is defined as an unexpected death of a baby during pregnancy, labour or following birth, and encompasses miscarriage, ectopic pregnancy, loss of a twin, stillbirth and neonatal death (Clark Callister 2006).

This experience of sudden loss may contrast to that experienced by parents and families when the child's death is expected, such as following a long-term chronic illness. Rando (1986) suggests that parents may have more time to anticipate the loss and begin their grieving and that this may have a positive impact on their coping following the loss. When individuals are faced with the likelihood of a significant loss, they may embark upon the process of anticipatory grief (Fulton et al. 1996).

Anticipatory grief refers to commencement of the grieving process prior to the anticipated loss and may have positive outcomes, as it enables people to begin to work through the changes surrounding the loss and therefore lessens the trauma experienced when the loss occurs. However, whether anticipatory grief actually lessens the impact of the loss once it occurs is the subject of debate in bereavement literature (Walker et al. 1996). It should never be assumed that when a death was anticipated that it will be less painful than a sudden death, or that grieving will be a less difficult process. In fact, it is suggested that in some situations where caregiving has led to other problems or a relationship is dependent or guilt-ridden, the grief can be intense (Brazil et al. 2002). In addition to anticipatory grief, parents, the child and family members are likely to have been on a journey punctuated by painful procedures, therapies and surgery in an effort to cure or enhance quality of life, periods of hope, loss of hope and cycles of relapse, remission and relapse (Rando 1986).

The relationship between the child, their family and health professionals in the long-term care situation will also contrast to the context of sudden unexpected death. In the former case, relationships may have developed over a long period of time and opportunities may have arisen to instigate bereavement support much earlier and offer it more constantly and consistently prior to the child's death.

Grief within the context of the family

In the context of child, youth and family nursing, it is essential to understand developmental differences in responses to loss. When loss occurs, it impacts on all members of the family. In the case scenario, the loss of baby Julie has impacted on the parents Jacqui and Mark, as well as their children, Alex and John, in unique ways. To explore your understanding so far, refer to the critical reflections and questions in Box 11.1.

Box 11.1 Critical reflections and questions: responses to grief

Following your reading in the chapter so far and reflection on the case scenario, discuss how the following factors could influence the grief response for each of the family members:

1. their age and developmental stage
2. their gender
3. history of the loss/trauma
4. the nature and quality of the relationship with the deceased, and
5. the circumstances surrounding the loss (e.g. anticipated or sudden unexpected, traumatic, and family relationships and expectations).

Loss is both a personal and an interactional process that occurs within a social context where people grieve within personal, family and societal systems (Neimeyer 2000).

People's values and expectations may assert their influence on the experience of grief in subtle or overt ways. In some cases of perinatal loss, there may be powerful societal expectations concerning grieving and sometimes limited recognition of the family's need to grieve and hold rituals (Clark Callister 2006). The manner in which family, friends and acquaintances respond to grieving families, albeit well-intentioned, can sometimes deepen rather than ease the pain experienced following loss of a loved one (Shumaker & Brownell 1984). In the case scenario, consider how social networks and expectations may help or hinder Jacqui, Mark, Alex and John's grief.

Debate surrounding whether it is beneficial for parents to hold their stillborn baby continues. To understand this further, refer to the research highlight in Box 11.2.

Box 11.2 Research highlight: stillbirth—to hold or not to hold

Reynolds (2004), in his discussion about whether parents should hold or not hold their stillborn baby, reminds us that seeing or holding the deceased baby may be confronting for parents and 'may deprive them of the much needed protection of denial' (p. 87). However, he advocates an individualised rather than 'one size fits all' approach to psychosocial care of parents following stillbirth, where options are offered to parents along with an informed discussion of the risks and benefits. Such an approach acknowledges that 'patients have the right to absorb or not absorb the full reality of their loss . . . parents must face the reality of their loss on their own terms, not ours' (p. 87).

Loss of a child: parental grief

According to Rando (1986 p. 6):

> 'The loss of a child through death is quite unlike any other loss known . . . In comparison with other types of bereavement, the grief of parents is particularly severe, complicated and long lasting, with major and unparalleled symptom fluctuations occurring over time.'

Parents who have lost a child often say that their pain is so deep that it lasts a lifetime, despite their efforts to find meaning in life and move forward (Schwab 1997). The death of a child symbolises many social losses for parents whose focus and purpose had centred on nurturing their growth and development (Sanders 1986). Society holds the parents of successful children in high esteem and parents love and feel responsible for their children and believe that they will outlive them, their existence ensuring that parents retain a small sense of immortality (Sanders 1986).

When a child dies, parents can feel that they have failed their child and may become immersed in guilt and blame that may be directed towards themselves and their partners (Sanders 1986). Regardless of whether the child is young or an adult, or the death sudden or expected, the loss of a child is devastating, and shatters parental dreams, hopes, expectations, fantasies and wishes for that child (Rando 1986, Wheeler 2001, deJong-Berg & Kane 2006).

The grief of other children

There is considerable debate in the literature concerning the capacity of children to mourn. On one side, psychodynamic theorists, such as Wolfenstein (1966), Deutsch (1937) and Anna Freud (1960), argued that mourning was not possible until late childhood or adolescence. In contrast, John Bowlby's (1963, 1980) attachment theory argued that children as young as toddlers experienced grief reactions similar to those of adults. With respect to the attachment theory, it was argued that once a child was able to attach to another, they would mourn when that love object was removed. Other theorists (Furman 1964, Kliman 1989) have suggested a middle ground, arguing that children from 3 to 4 years of age are able to mourn.

The belief that children are not affected by loss is reinforced if children manifest grief differently from adults (Schwab 1997, Dyregrov 1990). While adults may display constant disturbance associated with the loss, some children do not cry, or continue to play as if nothing has happened (Schoen et al. 2004).

Mourning is not only experienced; it is also learned from those around the child. The child's environment will change when adults within that environment are mourning a situation, which can make the child feel insecure and stressed. Following the death of a child, parents may gain strength and purpose from their other children, while others find their own grief can leave them so depleted of emotional energy that they have difficulties supporting their children or partner (Boerner & Silverman 2001). The difficulty that some parents have of 'letting go' of the deceased child can lead to psychological pressure being placed on siblings to fulfil roles of the deceased child, or to take on characteristics of the deceased, a phenomenon often referred to as the 'replacement child' (Cain et al. 1964, Crehan 2004, Grout & Romanoff 2000). This psychological pressure can undermine the sibling's opportunities to live their own life and develop an individual identity. The child may be constrained by parental overprotection and restriction, or by being viewed as replacing the lost child (Crehan 2004, Grout & Romanoff 2000).

Aside from adults' individual functioning following loss and its effect on children and adolescents, the family system can give children some very strong messages about loss and how it is to be handled (Silverman et al. 1995). Often these messages are given subtly and largely unconsciously. However, children learn the patterns of acceptable behaviour very quickly. Family stories and meanings reconstructed in the context of loss of a child are conveyed to all surviving family members and have a strong influence on family practices as well as child development (Grout & Romanoff 2000).

Child development and bereavement

From conception to death, a human being is developing and changing. Innate and learned skills are used to adapt to the circumstances of our existence and the changes that are occurring around us. The major difference between adults and children is that children may be experiencing these demands on their abilities for the first time without the benefit of hindsight and the intellectual ability to 'think through' the changes, the options and their consequences in a logical manner. In addition, the intensity of change is more pronounced in the life of children than it is in the life of adults, as so many changes are occurring within a relatively short period of time from birth to adolescence.

For many children, these vast changes will occur within the security of a loving family environment. The changes will occur gradually, in line with the expectations of the supportive adults around them and in common with their peers. Children in these circumstances will likely develop positive coping skills, often mirroring the well-adjusted adults in their lives. However, many children will have to deal with the critical changes of childhood without these advantages. Into the lives of such children may come devastating loss that is out of the realm of experience of the adults around them, or that renders the adults emotionally unable to provide the necessary support and insight for the child. In other situations, the normal demands of change and the losses of life on the growing child are complicated by physical and intellectual difficulties with which the child is born, the negative physical environment in which they live, and/or the maladaptive behaviours of the adults around them.

In considering the development of the child, there has been a tendency to consider physical, intellectual, emotional and social development as separate influences. However, these developmental demands occur simultaneously, with children experiencing many changes within a relatively short period of time. Difficulties in one area alone will require children to draw on their resources. Difficulties in more than one area at the same time will tax those resources—maybe even overload them. Box 11.3 provides a summary of children's reactions to death.

So what might a child understand about death?

Grieving is a highly emotional time in the life of a family. Hence, children with limited expressive language like Alex who is 4 years old may find it more difficult to verbalise their feelings or concerns of an event.

A 10-year follow-up study into children's reactions to the perinatal death of a sibling by Murray (2005b) highlighted that the stage of development of the child at the time of death is a significant factor affecting the long-term outcomes of bereavement. One of the major differences in the grieving of children and adults is that children's grieving occurs within a child's world and they lack the experiences into which to 'fit' their situation of loss.

Baker et al. (1992) identified two important aspects of grieving in children: the need for protection, and the need to maintain an internal representation and relationship with the lost object. They argue that a failure to recognise the significance of these aspects may contribute to short-term and long-term problems in children. Burnell and Burnell (1989) suggest that there are three questions that concern children and need to be addressed in their understandings of what is happening around them:

1. 'What did I do to cause this to happen?'
2. 'Will this happen to me too? Or will something "bad" happen to me too?'
3. 'Who will take care of me?'

These questions can be linked to early childhood thinking, which is egocentric, magical and where cause and effect is poorly understood—that is, normal developmental behaviours (Hockenberry et al. 2003).

In relation to health and illness, young children may also be influenced by immanent justice, where they may believe they are at fault and that accidents

Box 11.3 Practice highlight: children's reactions to death

The summary below gives a few of the more important points about the understandings of death in children at different ages.

Infants

Infants:

- have no concept of death or time
- may not be able to form a permanent image of the object or person lost
- are mainly affected by their carer's emotional state, which may lead to a decreased ability on the part of the carer to provide for the needs of the baby or respond to the baby's needs or actions—as a result, the baby may become more 'fussy' or 'clingy', and
- one twin may be affected by loss of the other twin.

Toddlers and preschoolers

Young children have little understanding of the irreversible nature or permanence of some situations of loss, including death. A carer may explain the situation, only to find the child asking when the situation will return to normal. Saying that if someone is dead they will *never* come back may be quickly met with the question, 'But when will . . . come home?' Death may only be thought of in terms of being 'not here' as opposed to being 'here'. Therefore, if someone is 'not here', you may be able to go and find them.

Young children may have difficulty distinguishing fact from fantasy. Therefore, the facts of the situation may be modified, changed or completely altered in the world of the imagination of the child. Separation anxiety is common. Fears are common. There may be intense searching for the person who has gone or died. Children may pull away from people who remind them too much of the person they have lost.

Prelogical thinking can lead to misconceptions or misinterpretations of what is said. 'Magical', egocentric thinking can lead them to believe that they have control over the outcome of a situation or were in some way responsible for the loss by some thought or action on their part.

Young children are often very curious about facts. They may not understand that, in death, the functions of life have ceased. Therefore, they may be concerned about a person being hungry, cold or breathing once buried. A lack of understanding of the consequences of a loss may result in a lack of reaction to news of the loss, which may be disconcerting to older children and adults.

Three most painful grieving emotions of the under 3s are likely to be:

1. separation fear—the ever-present fear that they will be abandoned by those they love
2. ambivalence—children's uncertainty about whether or not they should become attached to someone, and
3. guilt and hostility resulting from a child feeling responsible for the death or the distress in the family (Salladay & Royal 1981).

Very young children's grief may revolve around three questions:

1. 'What is death?'
2. 'Can it happen to me?'
3. 'Can it happen to you?' (Furman 1964).

cont.

Box 11.3 Practice highlight: children's reactions to death—*cont.*

Early school age

Children at this age are beginning to understand consequences. Therefore, they may have very definite opinions about causes of a loss. They may be very sure about what caused the death and place very definite blame on a particular person, even if it is not justified. In fact, in their fantasies they can take revenge on this person. These children may also believe strongly that if certain actions are carried out, they can avoid consequences. They may even fantasise that they can change the situation by these actions. Problems arise when the child has misconceptions concerning the causes of a loss. Issues of justice and injustice begin to emerge.

Children of this age are beginning to understand that loss affects others and can understand others' perspectives to some extent. They may try to sort out their ideas through playing out a situation. Therefore, concrete expressions such as rituals and drawing can support coping with loss.

Children of this age are gradually beginning to understand that death happens to everyone, but not themselves initially. Socialisation is becoming important (e.g. boys may begin to hide their feelings). However, isolation from peers after loss is common at this age. Children of this age can begin to plan and develop more coping strategies. An ability to plan may help to make a child feel more in control of their situation and their life in general.

Late school age/adolescence

Adolescents develop a mature understanding of death. Fear of death may come with this understanding. As a result of this fear, adolescents may try to keep these thoughts at a distance. Adolescents may also develop a personification of death. The four main types of death personification are the macabre (decaying form), the gentle comforter (powerful force quietly employed in a kindly way), the gay deceiver (luring in the unwary and leading them to their doom) and the automaton (goes about the business of death in a bored competent fashion) (Cotter 2003).

The need to deal with loss may be complicated by normal crises of adolescence. For example, at a time when parental support may be vital in dealing with a loss, the adolescent may be struggling with the issues and inevitable conflicts of wanting to be independent from parents.

At this stage, peer support is important. Unfortunately, many adolescents faced with a loss can feel their friends 'just don't understand'. At times, adolescents will deal with their sense of helplessness by engaging in 'risky' behaviour (e.g. experimenting with drugs, increased sexual activity, fast driving). Adolescents may also be very judgmental. They can be very hard on themselves if they believe they could have done more to prevent a loss. They may also become very angry with others they perceive to have some responsibility for the loss.

Shame plays an important part in adolescents' feelings of loss. Feelings or types of loss that an adolescent considers embarrassing or 'shameful' may be hidden. Paradoxically, the more intense the emotions an adolescent feels, the more they may try to repress them. The adolescent, particularly a boy, may be very fearful of losing control of their emotions. They may resist any attempts to get them to 'open up'. This conflict may appear in behaviour and conflicts with others in their environment.

or illness are magically caused by their own disobedience or misbehaviour, even though it was unconnected to the injury or illness (Raman & Winer 2004). A young child's belief in immanent justice can manifest in a variety of ways. For example, if someone says 'if you keep doing that, you'll be the death of me' and then they happen to die soon after, the child may think they have caused the death of that person (Schaefer & Lyons 1993). These cognitive distortions concerning death and their own contribution are exacerbated by lack of opportunity to talk about death and ask questions (Schwab 1997). For further exploration of these ideas, refer to Box 11.4.

Box 11.4 Critical questions and reflections: talking to children about death

When talking to children, it is important to be honest and use language to which the children can relate. It is also important to use the correct words to describe what is occurring (such as 'dead'). If children do not have information, they will often make something up to fill the gaps. This may be more damaging for them in the long term than knowing the truth if their interpretations of the event are incorrect. Tell the children that it is okay for them to feel sad, mad, angry or scared—to feel whatever it is that they need to feel or how they need to be.

It is very important to hear from and listen to the children to find out what they have heard or understood. Sometimes, children will hear part of what you say and 'close down' after hearing a single word or sentence. This is where misunderstanding can occur. Hence, try to help confirm that the children have heard and understood what you have tried to tell them, and gently encourage them to tell back to you what you told them. You may need to revisit these issues a few times to confirm understanding, but do not push too hard.

You are the midwife caring for Jacqui. She asks you how she should explain Julie's death to her children, particularly 4-year-old Alex. Discuss how you would suggest she explain Julie's death to her preschool-aged child.

The young child does not understand the irreversibility of death and may think that if they wish hard enough the person will return (Schaefer & Lyons 1993). They may not understand where their playmate has gone or may wonder why their parents have changed so much. Young children may also take adults' comments literally. For example, the comment 'your grandpa died so peacefully in his sleep' may result in the child not wanting to go to sleep for fear it will happen to them (Schaefer & Lyons 1993).

Most researchers agree that a child needs to understand three concepts of death as they mature. These concepts are:

1. *Universality/inevitability*: the understanding that all things die and that there is no avoiding it.
2. *Irreversibility*: the understanding that once a living thing dies, its physical body cannot be alive again.
3. *Non-functionality*: the understanding that all life-defining functions cease at death.

A comprehensive review of studies published since the 1980s concerning the conceptions of death among children (Kenyon 2001) led to the following conclusions:

- By 10 years of age, most children have mastered the components of irreversibility, universality, non-functionality, personal mortality and causality.

- Understanding these individual components appears to be differentiated by several factors, and appears to have different developmental trajectories.
- Abstract components such as universality appear to be affected by cognitive development, verbal ability, and cultural and religious experiences.
- Physical-based components such as non-functionality and irreversibility appear to be affected by direct experience.
- Emotional factors appear to play a significant role in how children respond to questions about death and might be highly influential in the development of their understanding about death.

A child's grief reaction will depend on their developmental stage. Burnell and Burnell (1989) suggest that children under 3 in families in which death has occurred will typically exhibit loss of speech and generalised distress, while children under 5 may respond with disturbances in eating, sleeping, bladder and bowel control. In school-age children, school phobias, hypochondriacal concerns (fear of being 'sick' or phantom illnesses), abdominal or substernal pain or headaches without organic origin, learning problems, antisocial behaviour, aggression or withdrawal are common responses. Grief reactions among older children may be more diverse than are those among younger children whose world of experience and repertoire of behaviours is more limited.

The older sibling in the case scenario, John, is 14 years old. By the time children enter adolescence, most have developed the ability to understand loss from the perspective of adults (Geis et al. 1998, Speece & Brent 1992). They are able to understand what has occurred and the short-term and long-term implications of the situation. As intellectual and emotional development occurs, children can need to reprocess aspects of a previous experience to deepen their understanding of the event (Schoen et al. 2004). The effects of loss in the lives of children or adolescents cannot be easily segregated from normal developmental changes. Adolescents are likely to understand as adults what happens when someone dies, as they now see death as universal, inevitable and irreversible (Schaefer & Lyons 1993).

Adolescents may express their grief through aggression, anger, withdrawal, anxiety including panic attacks, truancy, delinquency, fixation with the lost object, work or study deterioration, confusion, inappropriate laughter, hysteria, denial or guilt. However, they may also display physical symptoms such as nausea (Smith et al. 1988).

Providing supportive care to families

> 'Suffering is not a question that demands an answer;
> It is not a problem that demands a solution;
> It is a mystery that demands a presence.'—Anon

Nurses and midwives are socialised into a model of clinical decision making that includes assessment, identification of problems, planning and evaluating interventions. This clinical decision-making process underscores nurses' everyday actions and in the context of loss and grief may lead to a tendency to want to 'intervene' or resolve. However, this is inappropriate, as the loss is irreversible, and the problem cannot be resolved. The focus shifts, therefore, to interactions with families that are helpful and do not worsen an already overwhelming and deeply sad experience.

The loss experienced cannot be understood. However, it can be acknowledged by a sincere, simple and personalised expression of sorrow. Responses to siblings are guided by an understanding of their developmental level and understanding of death (see Box 11.3) and in the midst of parental grief it is important to be sensitive to sibling needs, questions and reactions to seeing others around them expressing grief. It is important to be aware that children may not interpret or understand what is happening in the same way in which adults do.

Nurses and midwives are often present within the intimate family circle at the time of loss, and may be uncertain about what to say. You will at times be a supportive presence for families where no words are necessarily spoken. However, when you do speak you can verbalise your thought processes to parents simply and honestly. A useful strategy here is to listen to your thoughts at the time you are approaching or sitting with a bereaved family. What are you thinking? Your thoughts may include: 'This is the worst experience imaginable, I can't imagine what you must be going through right now, I don't know what to say, I don't want to make things worse for you right now.'

The next step is to turn these thoughts into communication with the bereaved family: 'I was on my way here and I was thinking that this must be the most heartbreaking experience you could ever face. I can't imagine what you must be going through right now, but I want you to know that I want to do anything I can so as not to make this experience any worse for you right now.'

Lastly, nurses and midwives can personalise the child by talking to parents about their child and the memories they mention. By talking with parents you are recognising their incredible loss, acknowledging that they have lost someone so precious, along with all the hopes, dreams and future moments and milestones they wanted to share with their child.

Conclusion

In this chapter, you have considered definitions of grief and loss, reviewed current trends in thinking in relation to grief and loss, and through the critical thinking questions have had the opportunity to reflect upon the variety of factors that impact on parents and children and their responses to loss in the realm of child health nursing practice. An understanding of the myriad factors that influence individuals and their responses to grief is invaluable in providing sensitive and supportive care in this context.

Practice tips

- Acknowledge and validate the person's loss.
- Verbalise your thought processes to parents simply and honestly.
- Personalise the parents' child.

Useful resources

Australian Centre for Grief and Bereavement: www.grief.org.au/.
Australian Government Department of Health and Ageing: www.health.gov.au/internet/wcms/publishing.nsf/Content/palliativecare-pubs-rsch-grief.
Childhood Bereavement Centre at Mt Olivett: www.childbereavement.org.au.
Compassionate Friends: www.thecompassionatefriends.org.au/TCFAustralia.htm.
GriefLink: www.grieflink.asn.au/frameset.html.
NALAG: www.nalag.org.au.
SANDS: www.sands.org.au.
SIDS and KIDS: www.sidsandkids.org.

References

Baker JE, Sedney MA, Gross E 1992 Psychological tasks for bereaved children. *American Journal of Orthopsychiatry* 62(1):105–16.

Boerner K, Silverman PR 2001 Gender specific coping patterns in widowed parents with dependent children. *Omega: The Journal of Death and Dying* 43(3):201–16.

Bonanno G, Kaltmann S 1999 Toward an integrative perspective on bereavement. *Psychological Bulletin* 125:760–76.

Bowlby J 1961 Process of mourning. *International Journal of Psychoanalysis* 42:317–40.

Bowlby J 1963 Pathological mourning and childhood mourning. *Journal of the American Psychoanalytic Association* 11:500–41.

Bowlby J 1980 *Attachment and loss: loss, sadness and depression*. Basic Books, New York.

Brazil K, Bėdard M, Willison K 2002 Correlates of health status for family caregivers in bereavement. *Journal of Palliative Medicine* 5:849–55.

Burnell GM, Burnell AL 1989 *Clinical management of bereavement: a handbook for healthcare professionals*. Human Sciences Press, New York.

Cain AC, Fast I, Erickson ME 1964 Children's disturbed reactions to the death of a sibling. *American Journal of Orthopsychiatry* 34:741–52.

Calhoun LG, Tedeschi RG 2006 *Handbook of posttraumatic growth: research and practice*. Lawrence Erlbaum Associates Publishers, Mahwah, New Jersey.

Clark Callister L 2006 Perinatal loss: a family perspective. *Journal of Perinatal and Neonatal Nursing* 20(3):227–34.

Cotter RP 2003 High risk behaviours in adolescence and their relationship to death anxiety and death personifications. *OMEGA: The Journal of Death and Dying* 47(2):119–37.

Crehan G 2004 The surviving sibling: the effects of sibling death in childhood. *Psychoanalytic Psychotherapy* 18(2):202–19.

Davis CG, Wortman CB, Lehman DR, Silver RC 2000 Searching for meaning in loss: are clinical assumptions correct? *Death Studies* 24:497–540.

deJong-Berg MA, Kane L 2006 Bereavement care for families part 2: evaluation of a pediatric follow-up programme. *International Journal of Palliative Nursing* 12(10):484–94.

Deutsch H 1937 Absence of grief. *Psychoanalytic Quarterly* 6:12–22.

Doka KJ 1989 *Disenfranchised grief: recognizing hidden sorrows*. Lexington Books, Lexington.

Dyregrov A 1990 Children's reactions to grief and crisis situations. In A Dyregrov (ed.), *Grief in children: a handbook for adults*. Jessica Kingsley, London, pp. 9–28.

Freud A 1960 Discussion of Dr John Bowlby's paper. *Psychoanalytic Study of the Child* 15:53–63.

Freud S 1917 Mourning and melancholia. In *Sigmund Freud, Collected papers*, Vol. 4. Hogarth Press, London.

Fulton G, Madden C, Minichiello V 1996 The social construction of anticipatory grief. *Social Science and Medicine* 43(9):1349–58.

Furman R 1964 Death and the young child: some preliminary considerations. *Psychoanalytic Study of the Child* 19:321–33.

Geis HK, Whittlesey SW, McDonald NB et al. 1998 Bereavement and loss in childhood. *Child and Adolescent Psychiatric Clinics of North America* 7(1):73–85.

Genevro JL, Marshall T, Miller T 2004 Report on bereavement and grief research. *Death Studies* 28(6):491–575.

Glick I, Weiss RS, Parkes CM 1974 *The first year of bereavement*. Wiley, New York.

Grout LA, Romanoff BD 2000 The myth of the replacement child: parents' stories and practices after perinatal death. *Death Studies* 24:93–113.

Hockenberry M, Wilson D, Winkelstein M, Kline NE 2003 *Wong's nursing care of infants and children*, 7th edn. Mosby, St Louis.

Iserson KV 2000 Notifying survivors about sudden, unexpected deaths. *Western Journal of Medicine* 173:261–5.

Janoff-Bulman R 1992 *Shattered assumptions: towards a new psychology of trauma*. The Free Press, New York.

Kenyon B 2001 Current research in children's conception of death: a critical review. *OMEGA: The Journal of Death and Dying* 43(1):69–91.

Kliman G 1989 Facilitation of mourning during childhood. In SC Klagsburn, GW Kuman, EJ Clark & AH Kutscher et al. (eds), *Preventive psychiatry*. Charles Press, Philadelphia, pp. 59–82.

Kübler-Ross E 1969 *On death and dying*. MacMillan, New York.

Miller ED, Omarzu J 1998 New directions in loss research. In JH Harvey (ed.), *Perspectives on loss: a sourcebook*. Brunner/Mazel, Philadelphia, pp. 3–20.

Murray JA 2005a *A psychology of loss: a potentially integrating psychology for the future study of adverse life events. Advances in psychological research*, Vol. 37. Nova Publishers, New York, pp. 15–46.

Murray J 2005b Children's reactions to perinatal death of a sibling: a ten-year follow-up. Proceedings of the 2004 Mental Health Services Inc. of Australia and New Zealand Conference, Gold Coast, 1–3 September 2004, pp. 81–6.

Neimeyer RA 2000 *Lessons of loss: a guide to coping*. Centre for Grief Education, Victoria.

Neimeyer RA, Mahoney MJ (eds) 1995 *Constructivism in psychotherapy*. American Psychological Association, Washington DC.

Parkes CM 1972 *Bereavement: studies of grief in adult life*. International Universities Press, New York.

Parkes CM 1975 What becomes of redundant world models? A contribution to the study of adaptation to change. *British Journal of Medical Psychology* 48:131–7.

Parkes CM 1988 Bereavement as a psychosocial transition: processes of adaptation to change. *Journal of Social Issues* 44:53–65.

Raman L, Winer GA 2004 Evidence of more immanent justice responding in adults than children: a challenge to traditional developmental theories. *British Journal of Developmental Psychology* 22:255–74.

Rando TA 1986 *Parental loss of a child*. Research Press, Illinois.

Rando TA 1993 *Treatment of complicated mourning*. Research Press, Illinois.

Raphael B 1984 *The anatomy of bereavement: a handbook for the caring professions*. Hutchinson, London.

Reynolds JJ 2004 Stillbirth: to hold or not to hold. *OMEGA: The Journal of Death and Dying* 48(1):85–8.

Salladay SA, Royal ME 1981 Children and death: guidelines for grief work. *Child Psychiatry and Human Development* 11(4):203–12.

Sanders CM 1986 Accidental death of a child. In TA Rando, *Parental loss of a child*. Research Press, Illinois.

Schaefer D, Lyons C 1993 *How do we tell the children? A step-by-step guide for helping children two to teen cope when someone dies*. Newmarket Press, New York.

Schoen AA, Burgoyne M, Schoen SF 2004 Are the developmental needs of children in America adequately addressed during the grief process? *Journal of Instructional Psychology* 31(2):143–8.

Schwab R 1997 Parental mourning and children's behaviour. *Journal of Counselling and Development* 75:258–65.

Shumaker SA, Brownell A 1984 Toward a theory of social support: closing conceptual gaps. *Journal of Social Issues* 40(4):11–36.

Silverman PR, Weiner A, El Ad N 1995 Parent–child communication in bereaved Israeli families. *OMEGA: The Journal of Death and Dying* 31(4):275–93.

Smith GG, O'Rourke DF, Parker PE et al.1988 Panic and nausea instead of grief in an adolescent. *Journal of the American Academy of Child and Adolescent Psychiatry* 27(4):509–13.

Speece MW, Brent SB 1992 The acquisition of a mature understanding of three components of the concept of death. *Death Studies* 16:211–29.

Stroebe M, Schut H 1999 The dual process model of coping with bereavement: rationale and description. *Death Studies* 23:197–224.

Walker RJ, Pomeroy EC, McNeil JS, Franklin C 1996 Anticipatory grief and AIDS: strategies for intervening with caregivers. *Health and Social Work* 21(1):49–64.

Wheeler I 2001 Parental bereavement: the crisis of meaning. *Death Studies* 25:51–66.

Wolfenstein M 1966 How is mourning possible? *Psychoanalytic Study of the Child* 21:3–123.

Worden JW 1991 *Grief counseling and grief therapy: a handbook for the mental health practitioner*, 2nd edn. Tavistock/Routledge, London.

Wortman CB, Silver RC 2001 The myths of coping with loss revisited. In MS Stroebe, RO Hansson, W Stroebe & H Schut (eds), *Handbook of bereavement research: consequences, coping, and care*. American Psychological Association, Washington DC, pp. 405–29.

Chapter 12

Children with chronic health problems and their families

Jon Darvill, Kay Thomas and Pamela Henry

Learning outcomes

Reading this chapter will help you to:

- » identify common chronic health problems in Australia and New Zealand
- » describe the epidemiological incidences and trends of these health problems
- » identify the role of primary healthcare in their management
- » recognise that children themselves have a perspective on their lives, health and nursing care
- » reiterate in broad terms the best practice management approach to children with chronic health problems and their families
- » identify issues around the transition from paediatric to adult-based services
- » integrate current research findings into your nursing practice
- » adopt a culturally sensitive approach to nursing care of children and families with differing cultural practices
- » discuss the additional needs and challenges facing technology-dependent children and their families
- » describe issues around the preparation for and discharge of technology-dependent children from hospitals, and
- » identify the issues surrounding the provision of high levels of nursing care in the family home.

Introduction

Chronic diseases produce symptoms and develop over a long period of time. They are often complex and account for significant illness, disability and death in developed countries. O'Halloran et al. (2004) suggest that a chronic disease lasts at least 6 months, recurs or deteriorates, has a poor prognosis and the consequences of the disease impact on the individual's quality of life. Chronic diseases only emerged as population health problems in the twentieth century when significant control over infectious disease was achieved. They have now assumed epidemic proportions (Australian Institute of Health and Welfare 2006a). Finding effective solutions for individuals is, however, a complex challenge, as behaviour is contingent on many factors.

This chapter focuses on Australian and New Zealand children with chronic health problems and their families. It identifies the extent of these problems, their impact on children and families, and presents evidence of best practice management. The overarching assumptions encompassed in this chapter include the need to consider children and young people as individuals in their own right, adopt a primary healthcare approach, and promote collaborative models of care.

After discussing chronic health in children and young people, two clinical scenarios are used to introduce specific topics. Issues that are relevant not only to the specific scenario but also the wider population of chronically ill children and young people are discussed. The first scenario focuses on a young person with diabetes mellitus and the second is an infant who is dependent on technology for her survival.

Chronic health problems in children and young people

Chronic diseases in children and young people differ from those in adulthood in several ways, including their risk factors, incidence, and types and presentation of diseases. Chronic disease is predominantly seen in adults, but there is a smaller and significant number of children with long-term health problems. In 2001, 4% of New Zealand children had a chronic health problem and 3% had a psychiatric or psychological problem (Ministry of Health New Zealand 2004). In Australia, 41% of children suffer from a long-term problem, although this included relatively minor conditions such as those associated with vision (Australian Institute of Health and Welfare 2006b), which explains the wide discrepancy in statistics. Importantly, a chronic disease in a child affects not only the child, but also their family.

The chronic diseases responsible for the greatest disease burden in children differ from those in adults. Rather than coronary artery disease, stroke and chronic obstructive pulmonary disease (COPD), available data show that in both Australia and New Zealand childhood asthma, diabetes and cancer are responsible for a significant disease burden (Australian Institute of Health and Welfare 2005b, Ministry of Health New Zealand 1998). New Zealand also cites oral health as a significant issue. Other children's chronic conditions include, but are not limited to, cystic fibrosis, cerebral palsy, epilepsy, learning disabilities, visual impairment, allergies and the consequences of injury. Psychosocial health issues include conditions such as depression/anxiety, attention deficit hyperactivity disorder (ADHD) and autism.

Epidemiological data have identified several patterns or trends. While the incidences of asthma and cancer are not changing, the incidence of both type 1 and type 2 diabetes mellitus is rising. Type 2 is usually seen in people over 40 years of age and is associated with obesity and a sedentary lifestyle, both modifiable risk factors (Australian Institute of Health and Welfare 2005b). Lifestyle risk factors for developing adult chronic diseases persist in children and young people. Of particular concern is that the proportion of children and young people whose weight is unhealthy is rising. Finally, there are no discernible trends in mental health problems. Table 12.1 sets out the areas of concern and associated issues for chronic diseases in both Australia and New Zealand.

Chronic childhood health problems have differing patterns of presentation. Some are congenital, some develop later in life and some the child 'grows out of'. Despite this, most require healthcare to enable the child to live a normal or near normal life (Australian Institute of Health and Welfare 2005b).

Risk factors for developing the classic chronic health problems of adulthood can occur in childhood. Some risk factors occur early in life and are unique to childhood. See Table 1.1 in Chapter 1 for a summary of risk and protective factors. For example, a low birth weight (<2500 g) increases the risk of some cardiac, respiratory, renal diseases and type 2 diabetes (Australian Institute of Health and Welfare 2006b). Other risk factors are similar to those of adults and include individual, family and community factors.

Having outlined the major diseases and their incidence in childhood, it is worth personalising these data by considering the first of the two scenarios, which concerns a young person with a chronic disease and her family.

Scenario one: Josie—a young person with a chronic disease

Josie has just turned 13 years old. She presents to the Emergency Department with her 15-year-old sister, Michelle. Josie says she is feeling really tired and has been 'vomiting'. The triage nurse begins an assessment and during the history taking discovers Josie has a history of type 1 diabetes mellitus. Type 1 is the more common in children and young people and is characterised by the need for insulin replacement. It is an autoimmune disease, has no known modifiable risk factors (Australian Paediatric Endocrine Group 2005) and is the fastest growing health problem in this age group (Australian Institute of Health and Welfare 2005b).

Josie is diagnosed with diabetic ketoacidosis (DKA) and has 5% dehydration. She is rehydrated, treated with insulin and admitted to the Paediatric High Dependency Unit (HDU). During her admission, she is seen by the paediatric endocrinologist, diabetes educator, nutritionist and social worker.

Josie is experiencing an acute exacerbation of a chronic disease. While she requires hospitalisation and acute care now, this is a short interlude in her ongoing primary healthcare management. How Josie came to develop DKA and the fact that she presented with her sister rather than a parent are specific areas of concern for her health professionals. These may indicate she is having trouble at home.

Table 12.1 Health problems in Australia and New Zealand

Prevalence and trends	Key points
Diabetes mellitus *Australia* Type 1 (0–14 years old) 24.6/100,000 Increasing annually by 3% Type 2 is also increasing and accounts for 5% of all diabetics (Australian Institute of Health and Welfare 2005b) *New Zealand* Type 1 (0–14 years old) 14.7/100,000 Increasing incidence (Ministry of Health New Zealand 1998) Type 2 (10–14 years old) Maori 6.9/100,000; 92% were obese Increasing incidence (Campbell-Stokes & Taylor 2005)	Control of blood glucose levels (BGL) reduces the risk of complications common in adulthood. Most centres are currently not achieving target levels of HbA_{1c} (blood test used to monitor BGL over time). The optimal HbA_{1c} target is 7.5% or less without increasing hypoglycaemia. Early signs of long-term complications (retinopathy and increased albumen excretion rate) are common in children 6 years after diagnosis (Donaghue et al. 2005). Immediate concerns in childhood are lower quality of life, psychological problems and difficulty adjusting to adulthood (Ambler et al. 2006). Asymptomatic hypoglycaemia is more common than previously thought. It may cause neuropsychological damage in young children (Ambler et al. 2006).
Asthma *Australia* Little difference in prevalence between Indigenous and non-Indigenous children, but asthma is more prevalent in locally born children than those born overseas (Australian Institute of Health and Welfare 2005b) *New Zealand* (6–7 years old) 12-month prevalence of 26.5% (Asher et al. 2001)	*Australia* There is a strong link between asthma and allergy. 40% of children with asthma live with smokers (National Asthma Council 2006). Asthma was the most common reason for children's hospital admissions in 2003–04 and absence from school (Australian Institute of Health and Welfare 2005b). *New Zealand* Children's hospital admissions are approximately double that of adults. Maori and Pacific Islander children have lower usage rates of asthma medication, more severe symptoms and higher rates of hospitalisation (Asher & Byrnes 2006).
Cancer *Australia* Incidence of cancers is increasing on average by 0.6% per annum (Australian Institute of Health and Welfare 2005a, 2005b)	*Australia* Cancers are relatively rare compared with adults, with <1% of all cancers in 2001 occurring in children. Cancer is the leading cause of death in chronically ill children, causing 16% of all deaths in 2003. *cont.*

Table 12.1 Health problems in Australia and New Zealand—*cont.*

Prevalence and trends	Key points
Cancer—*cont.* *New Zealand* (0–14 years old) Prevalence of 16.51/100,000 in 2000–02 Second highest cause, after injury, of all deaths in this age group	Leukaemia and CNS cancers account for 57% of the new diagnoses in 2001 (Australian Institute of Health and Welfare 2005b). Improved survival to 5 years for children with leukaemia since the 1980s (62.4% to 69.7%). However, CNS malignancies remain a leading cause of death in this age group (Australian Institute of Health and Welfare 2006b). *New Zealand* Patterns are similar to Australia. The survival rate for children with brain tumours is far less impressive at a 25% 5-year survival.
Unhealthy weight *Australia* One in four children and adolescents is overweight or obese (Margarey et al. and Vaska et al., cited in Baur 2006) *New Zealand* In 2002, of children aged 5–14 years, 21.3% were overweight and 9.8% were obese The prevalence is generally greater among Pacific Islander and Maori populations than New Zealand Europeans and others (MOH 2006)	The epidemiological triad of obesity: 1. Host (the individual) Biological Behavioural Physical adjustments 2. Environment Physical, economic, policy, sociocultural 3. Vectors of obesity (factors that promote obesity): high-energy foods and drinks; labour-saving devices; and television and computers (Lean et al. 2006).
Smoking *Australia* Rates of smoking have halved over the last decade One in 12 young Australians aged 12–19 years smoked daily in 2004 (females 9.1%; males 7.3%) Declining number of households where someone is smoking inside (31% in 1995 to 12% in 2004) The number of households that include a smoker remains constant at 40–45% (Australian Institute of Health and Welfare 2006b) *New Zealand* Survey of secondary school students in 2000 By 13 years of age, 36.2% of males and 36.5% of females have smoked a cigarette 15 and 16 year olds are most likely to smoke cigarettes weekly or more	Smoking reduces health and fitness and increases the risk of lung cancer. This risk increases the younger the child starts smoking (Australian Institute of Health and Welfare 2006b). Passive smoking is associated with a variety of respiratory problems, including asthma and SIDS (Australian Institute of Health and Welfare 2006b). *cont.*

Table 12.1 Health problems in Australia and New Zealand—*cont.*

Prevalence and trends	Key points
Smoking—*cont.* Female students of all ages are more likely to smoke cigarettes than males (Adolescent Health Research Group 2003)	
Alcohol consumption *Australia* 1.7% of children between 12 and 14 years old are at risk of short-term problems and 0.4% are at risk of long-term consequences (Australian Institute of Health and Welfare 2006b) *New Zealand* Survey of secondary school students in 2000 >8 out of 10 students have drunk alcohol and most continue to do so >50% of student drinkers reported an episode of binge drinking (Adolescent Health Research Group 2004)	Alcohol health problems in children and adolescents relate to 'risky or binge' drinking (i.e. five or more drinks in one drinking session). This can lead to alcohol poisoning, accidents, violence and unprotected sex. Chronic problems such as addiction, organ damage, depression and relationship problems may occur (NDARC 2004, cited in Australian Institute of Health and Welfare 2006b). Chronic diseases, including cancers of the digestive system, cirrhosis of the liver, brain damage and fetal alcohol syndrome may occur (Adolescent Health Research Group 2004).
Illicit drugs (cannabis and others) *Australia* Surveys (2001 and 2002) of 12–19-year-old students and young people 27–38% used at least one illicit drug Cannabis: 25–34% prevalence. Use declined between 1993 and 2001 (Holt 2005) Other drugs (hallucinogens, amphetamines, cocaine, ecstasy, opiates and steroids): small proportion (<10%) report frequent use (Holt 2005) *New Zealand* Survey of secondary school students in 2000 Cannabis: at 16 years of age, about 50% of students of both sexes have tried cannabis. More frequent use is less prevalent (males 10.2%; females 8.3%) Other drugs: ecstasy, glue, hallucinogens, narcotics, stimulants or cocaine—reported use males 11.5%; females 11% (Adolescent Health Research Group 2003)	Cannabis is the most commonly used illicit drug. Illicit drug use is more common and may be normalised in specific subcultures (e.g. clubbing and dance music). Heroin use is stable at <1% of young people, but there is increasing use of recreational or party drugs such as ecstasy and amphetamines (Holt 2005).

Diagnosis and its impact on children and their families

Josie was diagnosed with diabetes mellitus at the age of 2 years. She was living with her mother, father and sister, Michelle, who was then 4 years old. For the family, Josie's diagnosis changed their lives. The diagnosis of a chronic illness signals the end of the known world for the family and its individual members. Uncertainty and a period in which the family attempts to adapt follow. Most families and children will strive to normalise their new situations (Fisher 2001, Knafl & Deatrick 2002, Darvill 2003). Some families are successful in their adaptation, while others are not and will remain vulnerable (Dellve et al. 2006). The ability to cope varies according to individual factors, the dynamics within the family and the specific health problem (Dellve et al. 2006).

The range of responses can be conceptualised as a continuum reflecting the difficulties the families have in their adaptation (Hentinen & Kyngas 1998, Knafl & Deatrick 2006), whether individuals' experiences are similar or different (Knafl & Deatrick 2006) and the degree of stability within the parenting relationship (Darvill 2003). Families often struggle with the emotional impact, the additional stress that is encountered and the loss of important aspects of their lives. Thus, stress arises from multiple sources—intrinsic, family, the child and from interactions with health services (Krulik et al. 1999, Chesla & Rungreangkulkiji 2001, Melnyk et al. 2001, Australian Institute of Health and Welfare 2005b, Dellve et al. 2006, Barlow & Ellard 2006).

Josie's mother and father were shocked at the diagnosis of a chronic disease requiring complex management. They watched their child suffer while undergoing medical treatment. They had to perform painful procedures such as blood glucose monitoring and injections of insulin themselves. Further, they lost a certain freedom in their lives as a new regime was required to manage Josie's diabetes.

The emotional impact is often ongoing with peaks of intensity at critical moments, such as if the child is not achieving a developmental milestone, transitional times including starting school and puberty or when the child is having an acute exacerbation related to their condition (Melnyk et al. 2001). Barlow and Ellard (2006) found that 5 years from diagnosis, the parents experience a range of issues. They may be fearful and uncertain or even display symptoms of post-traumatic stress. They are also likely to worry about their child's future and health. In contrast, some reviews they evaluated noted positive outcomes such as good support systems, the development of new values and attitudes, and increased bonding within marital relationships and families.

Parents are not the only ones who suffer. The children, both those with a chronic disease and their siblings, may also suffer, although again the evidence is inconsistent or incomplete. In addition to the consequences of the disease itself, the affected child is at a slightly higher risk of a psychosocial problem. The child may have difficulty adjusting to their circumstances, miss school, lose touch with friends and therefore risk social isolation. Thus the child may feel different, anxious and depressed, and may develop emotional and/or behavioural problems. The child's self-concept and self-esteem may be lower, although the evidence is again not consistent. The risk factors for developing these problems are also not clear. This makes specifically targeted interventions difficult (Barlow & Ellard 2006).

Siblings may have similar psychosocial problems. The severity of the affected sibling's illness can be related to this, as can the sibling receiving less attention from their parent(s), or experiencing disruption to family plans or outings (Barlow & Ellard 2006). Once again the evidence is mixed.

It is clear that having a chronically ill child in the family has the potential to impact on the psychosocial wellbeing of the family as a whole. These multiple and complex issues increase the burden on health systems to be responsive and to promote the wellbeing of the child and family. It is also clear that there are inconsistencies in the evidence, and in order to improve services there is a need for further rigorous research (Barlow & Ellard 2006).

Normalising and family management styles

An important goal of parents and children is normality (Fisher 2001, Knafl & Deatrick 2002, Darvill 2003). Normalisation is a dynamic process that changes over time, with some families normalising and others not. Normalisation entails two conceptual processes:

1. how individual members perceive their new situation, and
2. how they consequently manage the child (Deatrick et al. 1999).

Normalisation is seen in families who focus on the normal aspects of their child rather than focusing on what is different. This affects their management (Knafl & Deatrick 2006), enables them to eventually see their lives as normal, and to manage the illness successfully (Deatrick et al. 2006).

The characteristics of not having achieved normalisation (see Table 12.2) can also be seen as barriers to normalisation. These arise from the subjective views of the parents, conflicting opinions of their situation or the work involved in complying with the treatment regime. Families may exhibit one or more of these barriers (Knafl & Deatrick 2002).

Families may adopt what Knafl et al. (1996) described as a family management style (FMS), which is more than just a strategy such as normalising. The FMS is the configuration formed by the family, their definitions of their situation, their management behaviours and their sociocultural contexts (Knafl et al. 1996). (See Box 12.1.)

The child's perspective

Until very recently the point of view or voice of children with chronic illness has been ignored. Historically, children's perspectives have not been sought by qualitative researchers for two reasons. First, they are vulnerable to exploitation and, second, they have been thought of as incapable of participation. In Chapter 4, a discussion of ethical principles, guidelines and practice concerning research with children and young people is presented. Children are vulnerable, but this is not a reason to exclude them from active engagement. As helpful as developmental theories have been, the division of a child's life into stages (Santrock 2004) has constantly forced comparisons between children and adults. It highlights what children are incapable of rather than what they can do. This could be called a deficit model of children (Woodgate 2001).

Table 12.2 The characteristics of normalisation

Characteristics of the normalised family	Characteristics of the family not normalised
The parents: • acknowledge the condition and its potential to threaten their lifestyle • adopt the normalcy lens (focusing on normal aspects) for defining child and family • engage in parenting behaviours and family routines that are consistent with the normalcy lens • develop a treatment regime that is consistent with the normalcy lens, and • interact with others based on the view of the child and family as normal	The parents: • emphasise the child as being different and that parenting has changed to accommodate a dramatically different view of the child • describe the illness as the major focus of family life • describe the illness as a source of conflict, and • describe the treatment regime as a significant burden entailing behaviours that make them different from other families

It is increasingly recognised that children are capable of communicating thoughts and feelings on their health and that they are in the best position to do so (Clements et al. 2006). Sartain et al. (2000) explored the experience of chronically ill children, their parents and health professionals. They found that the children (8–14 years old) were effective participants in research and their voices indicated that they were not a homogeneous group, but reacted to and coped with hospitalisation in different ways. Such findings must impact on nursing research and practice, and guide development that includes children in consultation and decision making regarding not only individual care but also potentially service planning and policy (Steinbeck & Brodie 2006, Australian Capital Territory Government 2004, Department of Health 2004). Look at the photograph and Box 12.2 and consider the potential this type of strategy offers children and young people to participate in their healthcare.

Box 12.1 Research highlight: the family management styles framework

The FMS framework is evidence-based and describes how the family manages both their family life and the child's health problems (Deatrick et al. 2006). It is based on a continuum of five management styles: Thriving, Accommodating, Enduring, Struggling and Floundering. Examples are:

- *The 'Thriving' style:* families are confident about their ability to manage both usual and unexpected demands; the treatment required is seen as proactive.
- *The 'Struggling' style:* there is parental conflict based on differing views of the child's illness and their expectations of each other (Deatrick et al. 2006).

A clinical assessment tool that will measure a family's response to a child's chronic illness is currently being developed. The aim of the tool is to provide a valid and reliable measure of the family's response to facilitate interventions that specifically address that family's needs. The tool is currently being field-tested (Knafl & Deatrick 2006).

Box 12.2 Critical questions and reflections: a Disability Aid Dog may improve independence

A 14-year-old girl who requires overnight ventilation initiated the trial use of a Disability Aid Dog to wake her in response to equipment alarms. The aim is to reduce the need for overnight respite/in-home care and to promote her independence. Look at the photograph. Imagine the ways in which the dog may be helpful, not only at night but also in her life more generally.

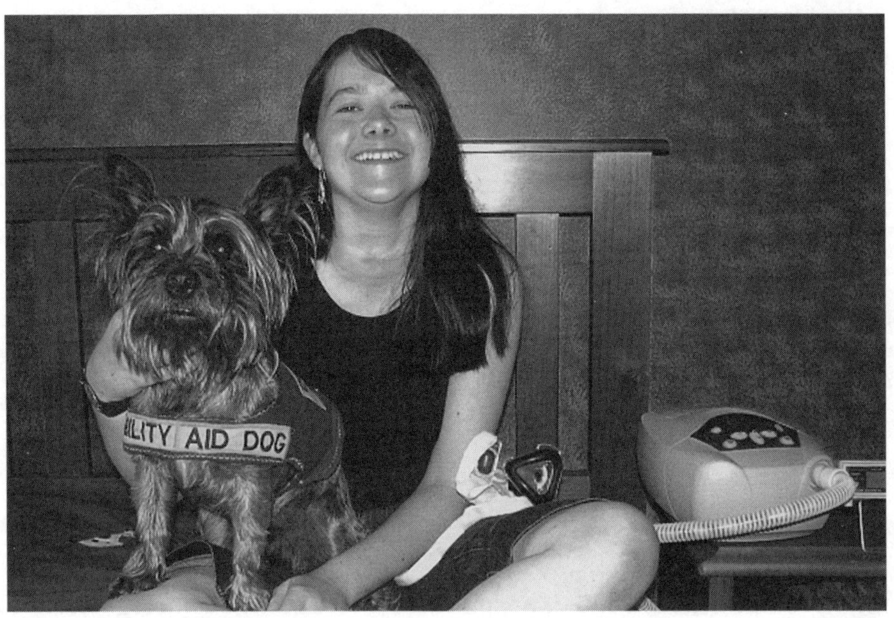

Adolescents: young people in transition

Josie is 13 years old. She, like other young people with chronic health problems, is in transition. She is somewhere between childhood and adulthood physically, emotionally and mentally. Over the next 5 years, she and other young people like her must also move on from the group of known health professionals to those in the unknown world of adult healthcare. These transitions are known to be difficult and problems arise frequently.

The diabetes educator speaks to Josie during her admission. The educator feels that the most likely cause of Josie's ketoacidosis is that she was not complying with her insulin administration.

Compliance with treatment regimes

Nurses historically understand compliance to mean adherence to medical advice. A more appropriate definition today is that the individual actively maintains their health in collaboration with the healthcare team (Kyngas & Rissanen 2001).

There could be many reasons why Josie was not administering enough insulin. These may relate to her knowledge of the drug. However, they may also relate to her motivation and self-management, and how the medication regime fits with her behaviours more generally (e.g. risk-taking behaviour or weight-loss schemes). The level of parental supervision may also be relevant.

It is estimated that 50% of young people with a chronic health problem do not comply with their treatment regime. However, being a young person in itself is not the issue, as non-compliance figures are similar in adults. Factors that promote compliance are well studied and those with a strong relationship to compliant behaviours include:

» good motivation
» a strong sense of normality
» a positive attitude towards the disease and treatment
» energy and willpower
» a subjective experience of results
» support from parents, friends, nurses and physicians, and
» a feeling that the condition was not a threat to one's social wellbeing (Kyngas 2000).

Predicting who is likely to comply and for what reasons is also important and is a focus of research. In a study of 300 adolescents (Kyngas & Rissanen 2001), compliance was predicted by several factors. Internal factors included the energy and the will to care for themselves and motivation. External factors included the support from nurses, parents, physicians and friends. Clearly, this is an important area for further research to develop practical tools for health professionals to use and to investigate ways to improve energy, will and motivation when necessary.

Moving from paediatric to adult services

Regardless of Josie's current problems, in a few years she will make the transition from the family-oriented and developmentally focused endocrinology healthcare team to more independently focused adult services. It is important that she, her family and her healthcare team begin planning now. Typically, transition can be a complex task and problems related to the lack of infrastructure, precedent and the preparedness of adult services are often encountered. Consequently, young people can remain in the care of paediatric/child health services longer than is desirable, move abruptly and in some instances disappear from the health services completely (Bennett et al. 2005).

Transition requires planning, on the part of the individual, their family, health professionals and policy makers. Nurses play an important role in advocating for their patients and preparing them for transition. There is an increasing number of transition programs being developed. One such program is the New South Wales Greater Metropolitan Clinical Taskforce Transition Care Program for Young People with Chronic Illness/Disability. The program was developed in 2002 after consultation with young people, their families and clinicians (Steinbeck & Brodie 2006). The program aims to ensure the young person:

1. exits paediatrics with a good understanding of their condition
2. demonstrates independent healthcare behaviour
3. is informed about the differences between paediatric and adult services, and
4. has begun to engage with their 'new' adult health service.

Transition programs in Australia and New Zealand are still developing and more research is needed, particularly around evaluation. However, Bennett et al. (2005) suggest that the most urgent need is for a change in health professionals' attitudes and approaches.

Our next scenario looks at Tihema, a Maori infant. This scenario focuses on children who are technology dependent. These children and their families face all the issues of chronicity, in addition to those related to the complexity of their health problems.

Scenario two: Tihema—a technology-dependent infant and her family

Tihema is 7 months post-term and has tracheomalacia, chronic lung disease and hypotonia. She has associated problems of acquired subglottic stenosis and feeding difficulty. She was born at 26 weeks gestation and required prolonged mechanical ventilation, as she was difficult to extubate. Tihema has a tracheostomy. She requires continuous positive airway pressure (CPAP) with supplementary oxygen when sleeping (some centres are now using variable (VPAP) or bi-level (BiPAP) respiratory machines) and gastrostomy feeding via a pump with a calorie supplemented infant formula, as she is not permitted to feed orally.

Her care is complex and a team of health professionals is working together to plan and deliver an holistic, individually designed program to support her needs and plan for her discharge.

Tihema's room is crowded with equipment and she is often restricted to her cot. Some photographs of family members are taped on her wall. A greenstone (taonga) is placed on the locker—a symbol of protection left by the family. Tihema has never been home.

Tihema's mother, Moana, is Maori. She lives in an urban area with high levels of deprivation. Moana has two other young children under 5 years old, and lives with her parents and three siblings. Moana is supported by her extended family. Her partner lives nearby. There have been incidents of domestic violence.

Developmental issues

In addition to her other problems, Tihema has been slow in achieving growth and developmental milestones. Babies and children who have complex health issues from an early age often have delayed developmental progress. The cause of the delay (neurological or environmental) may not be distinguishable until the child begins to improve in health and is discharged. These children are often restricted in their movement and in the time they are held and cuddled, normally because of physical instability and attachment to monitoring equipment. The balance between providing physical care and enhancing the achievement of milestones and family bonding is a significant challenge for both the family and the interdisciplinary health team.

A Maori model of health

For Maori, models of health are holistic. Durie's Whare tapa wha concept encompasses four dimensions. These include taha wairua (spiritual), taha hinengaro (mental), taha tinana (physical) and taha whanau (family). This concept of health requires an interaction of all these aspects, which represent four walls of a house. If one of these walls fails, the house will fall (Durie 1994). The challenge for nursing is to support the physical needs of the child within a culturally acceptable environment. In Chapter 3, issues for Maori health are discussed in more detail.

Technology-dependent children and young people

Children who are dependent on technology are defined as those '. . .who need both a medical device to compensate for the loss of a vital body function and substantial and ongoing nursing care to avert death or further disability' (Wagner et al., cited in Kirk 1998 p. 102). They are a:

> '. . . diverse group of children who vary according to the cause of illness, age of onset ranging from birth through to adolescence, duration (months to life long dependence), incidence and severity of associated disabilities, and frequency of using technology' (Glendinning et al. 2001 p. 323).

Children who are dependent on technology are a relatively new group being cared for in communities internationally, and in New Zealand and Australia. It is difficult to establish their precise number as data are not routinely collected centrally. However, they are significant users of health resources, disproportionally young (Glendinning et al. 2001) and increasing in numbers, particularly those requiring respiratory support (Edwards et al. 2003).

Some indication of the prevalence in Australia and New Zealand came from a survey of Australasian hospitals. The survey showed that of 199 children who met the inclusion criteria (extended length of stay, multiple admissions and admitted for respite care), 116 (58%) had a prolonged length of stay, 2 (1%) had been admitted for respite care, and 10.1% were 'living in hospital' because there was no suitable alternative. Aboriginal and Torres Strait Islander and Maori populations were overrepresented in the survey (Children's Hospitals Australasia 2005). There is a need to better identify these children in order to provide more appropriate support services and prevent further long-term inappropriate institutionalisation.

Most children dependent on technology are both chronically ill and reliant on a technological device. This suggests that there are both similarities and differences between these children and children who are chronically ill. They may be similar because of the sharing of a chronic health problem and different because of the addition of a technological device. Both groups encounter many of the same problems (see Table 12.3).

Going home

Tihema has been in hospital now for several months and discussions are in progress planning her referral to her home environment. The first transfer home with any

Table 12.3 Differentiating the impact of chronic disease and technology dependence

Issues	Reported for families with a chronically ill child	Reported for families with a technology-dependent child
Shock, emotional distress and stress	Yes	Yes
Uncertainty	Yes	Yes
Social disruption	Yes	Yes
Striving for normality	Yes	Yes
Struggles for control	Yes	Yes
Fragility of control	Yes	Yes
Loss of freedom	Yes	Yes
Problematic relationships	Yes	Yes
Poor physical and mental health	Yes	Yes
Problems with the provision of support and services	Yes	Yes
Financial burden	Yes	Yes
Positive benefits	Yes	Yes
Providing 24-hour care	No	Yes
Social isolation	No	Yes
Managing a technological device	No	Yes
Requiring carers	No	Yes
Homes/rooms become like ICUs	No	Yes
Multiagency nurse-led packages of services	No	Yes

technology-dependent child is usually the most difficult for families. Planning for the transfer home should commence early—that is, once the child is medically stable or as soon as it is known that the child will require long-term technological support. For Maori, important decisions are often made by the whanau (family). Therefore, Moana and her whanau were invited to a meeting with ward staff to prepare for Tihema's transfer home. Family member meetings such as this begin a process that enables the identification and management of specific and unique family issues.

Tihema will require 24-hour care when she goes home. The idea of organising respite or in-home care is raised at the whanau meeting because respite at home is not initially welcomed by Moana. This reaction is common (Mentro & Steward 2002, Miller 2002). Therefore, the advantages of support should be discussed. These include a discussion of the ways to reduce the burden of stress and preventing long-term institutional care. Discussion is also needed on the prevention of potential harm, while also enhancing family coping and sibling support, and providing opportunities for social interaction (Miller 2002, Neufeld et al. 2001). After some discussion within the whanau, there is agreement to access respite / in-home care.

A seven-step discharge planning process, predicated on case management, described by Boosfeld and O'Toole (2000) is useful in showing elements of the process that is needed to successfully transfer a child like Tihema to her home. The steps are:

1. needs assessment
2. identification of key workers
3. discharge proposal
4. interdisciplinary planning meetings
5. recruitment and selection of home-care teams
6. training, and
7. moving home.

Despite the difficult transition, going home is important. Children have the right to grow up in the family context, as families are considered the natural environment for growth and development (United Nations 1989). Care by families at home is therefore preferred (Stein 2001). The benefits are multifocal, including better health (e.g. through fewer infections) and better lifestyle through being part of a community and living in a nurturing environment with family members (Hewitt-Taylor 2005).

As the child makes the transition through the normal stages of growth and development, they may be able to take charge and gain a sense of control regarding their care. There are already a small number of young ventilator-dependent adults, who despite their challenges are succeeding in school, university, travel and have gained independence from their immediate families (Gilgoff & Gilgoff 2003).

Care programs helping to manage complexity

Following a transfer home, significant difficulties can be encountered. There may be housing problems and complex family social issues. Funding for home care and equipment may be difficult to obtain and it may be difficult to recruit carers/nurses. In addition, overall case management may be poor (Noyes 2002, Jardine & Wallis 1998).

Additional complexity can arise as many of the children and young people may also require disability, education, social and other support services in both the government and non-governmental sector (Noyes 2006b). Involving these services helps provide holistic child and family-centred care, as family needs should not solely be defined by their child's health needs, nor should the parent be seen as a nurse, but rather as a parent who is able to provide healthcare to the child as part of their overall needs (Murphy 2001). To address this complexity, individualised care packages can be used to bring together all the required services, such as the Family Choice Program outlined in Box 12.3.

To be cost effective and appropriate, care packages need to be carefully coordinated or case managed by interdisciplinary and multiagency teams in a collaborative approach. They need to provide access to services that are flexible and responsive, including short-term and long-term respite/in-home care and also to provide coordinated follow-up. These services need to be culturally appropriate, and ensure appropriate risk management and application of policies and standards (Noyes 2006b, Horsburgh & Trenholme 2002).

The best care packages are unlikely to succeed without a partnership being established between families and professionals. Partnerships that develop concepts of team effort, sharing of knowledge, respect, support and advocacy are important (Lindeke et al. 2002). Henry (2004) identified that parents valued the care continuity provided by a key worker and the community-based specialist paediatric nursing service. Home visits by the interdisciplinary team including a local primary paediatrician were extremely helpful in developing these partnerships. The families

Box 12.3 Practice highlight: the Family Choice Program

The Family Choice Program is one of a range of in-home and community-based services run by Home and Community Care from the Royal Children's Hospital, Melbourne, Victoria. The program provides home and community-based support to families of children with complex, ongoing health needs and frequent medical interventions. The key aim of the program is to facilitate the integration of these children into their community and prevent unnecessary admissions to hospital. It is state-wide and provides services to eligible children and young people aged between 0 and 17 years.

The Victorian Department of Human Services funds the program and it is the availability of this preexisting and coordinated funding which helps avoid the unnecessary delays in discharge commonly experienced if funding has to be sought on a case-by-case basis. The program adds to existing generic services and can be utilised to purchase respite care, carer training, medical consumables and equipment hire.

The program supports parents as the experts in the care of their child. It is based on partnerships between parents, the child's primary medical practitioner, a homecare nurse, a case manager and a diverse range of community service providers. Care is coordinated by a community case manager who links the partners. The manager undertakes an extensive, holistic assessment and works with the partners to develop a comprehensive plan of care and support based on the child's medical needs and the unique psychosocial circumstances of the child and their family.

Also pivotal to the program is the role of the homecare nurse, a registered nurse based at the nearest hospital with a paediatric service. In collaboration with the child's parents and primary medical practitioner, the nurse is responsible for the development of a written care manual and the training, monitoring and review of care workers in the home and other community settings. The homecare nurse provides the link between the acute medical and the home setting, and it is the maintenance of this link that is vital to ensure the child can be safely cared for in their community.

also appreciated those processes that supported planning and discussions relating to boundaries and role definition.

Tihema was transferred home significantly later than had been hoped for because of the complexity of funding formulas for equipment and accessing funds for carers. Less difficult was planning her access to preexisting services covering a range of specialists, such as a paediatric specialist homecare nursing service, Well Child/child health services, Maori health services, neurodevelopmental and speech therapy services, dietician and general practitioner.

Henry (2004) found that community-based paediatric services, especially within nursing, that transcend the boundaries of primary, secondary and tertiary settings help to reduce barriers encountered by families. (See Box 12.4.) These services are typical of what families with technology-dependent children may require in both New Zealand and Australia.

Funding home care

Tihema needs to go home with the same equipment that was used to maintain her in hospital. When transferring home any technology-dependent child or young

Box 12.4 Critical questions and reflections: planning safe discharge

You have received a referral to be involved in discharge planning for Tihema. The meeting is planned at the tertiary service. You represent local community services and have been asked to highlight the issues of caring for Tihema at home from a community perspective. Consider these under the themes:

- emotional support
- practical help, and
- information the family may need to ensure an effective discharge that sustains Tihema and her family at home.

Put together a list of local resources. Include ideas for accessing funding to facilitate development of a comprehensive package of care (including respite/in-home care), which can be in place before Tihema is discharged home.

person, there is the expense of purchasing equipment as well as ongoing costs such as administration, staff wages, equipment maintenance and single-use items. Care workers / professionals and family who will provide the respite / in-home care require training. Families will have individual and specific requirements. Respite / in-home staff need to be culturally aware and apply appropriate values in the home setting.

In Tihema's case, several family friends who live outside the home will be employed by an agency. In other cases, staff unknown to the family would be employed through the local health service or agency. Any respite / in-home carers should be matched with families as closely as possible, as the aim is to provide sustainable care that maintains family function.

Often tensions arise related to funding. For example, there is pressure to reduce length of stay in hospital because of the cost of admission and demand for beds. Accessing discharge funding for technology-dependent children in New Zealand is complex and revolves around eligibility criteria and government funding systems. There are documented concerns that access to funds has not been equitable and needs-based across New Zealand. Regional discussions are occurring nationally to address the issues (Baker 2003). In Australia, access to funding varies from state to state and can also be dependent on eligibility criteria or as part of an overall individual government-funded care package.

Technology dependence and families

Families with a technology-dependent child will face unique problems, including managing the technological device. The complexity varies, with some families facing the responsibility of caring for a child on life support, whereas others manage lower levels of technology. In addition, families confront additional challenges. Four are described below.

First is the impact of needing the technology. The impact on families has been described (see Table 12.3) and is beginning to be quantified. Noyes (2007) found that ventilator-dependent children reported lower quality of life scores on their health and in other domains than their friends and chronically ill children. Requiring a technological device may have a number of other impacts, each one significant and needing resolution. It may delay discharge from hospital (Noyes 2000), increase family spending (Glendinning et al. 2001), limit school, employment and social life because of the time required to manage the technology (Heaton et al. 2005), and turn homes or rooms into intensive care areas.

A recent qualitative ethnographic study exploring the perceptions and experiences of Maori families caring for their technology-dependent child found that the interrelating factors that impact on the child and their families are complex and there was a significant impact on the parents' health (Henry 2004). As with families with a chronically ill child, some families with a technology-dependent child develop strategies that maintain a functioning family and the relationships within by regularly using health and respite services and obtaining financial assistance as well as establishing a degree of privacy in their own home (Darvill 2003, O'Brien 2001). Other families live in a state of chaos, experiencing constant change and extreme suffering (Darvill 2003).

The second challenge is heeding the children's/young people's perspective. Children and young people themselves who are technology dependent are an emerging new group creating their own novel lifestyles (Noyes 2006a). They are able to give voice to their experiences and describe them in a way that is meaningful (Darvill 2003), and describe emotional deprivation and educational and social exclusion when services provided do not meet holistic needs (Noyes 2000).

They suffer anxiety, painful procedures, long periods of hospitalisation and being different (Darvill 2003). In one unstable family within Darvill's study, registered nurses and carers were obliged to take on a parenting role. This led to the child forming inappropriate attachments and experiencing additional emotional suffering when staff moved in and out of employment.

Regarding their own health, children and young people may be more positive than their parents and hold more positive attitudes towards their technology. British children felt better on the ventilator (Noyes 2006a). Canadian ventilator-dependent children described a major theme of 'It's okay. It helps me to breathe' (Earle et al. 2006). Darvill (2003) found some Australian children were growing up and doing normal things despite their health problems. They clearly understood their technology and were increasingly able to use it. Knowing the children's perspective is extremely important. It challenges professionals' understanding of the meaning of children's health and disabilities, concepts of what resources are needed to achieve a good quality of life (Noyes 2006a) and the ability to incorporate their point of view into nursing practice (Darvill 2003).

The third challenge focuses on incorporating technology in the family home. Families have to change to accommodate a technology-dependent child and their equipment within the home environment. Structural home modifications may be required before discharge. Other changes may include taking on the added role as administrators of complex regimes and providing highly technical clinical procedures that sometimes cause pain and suffering. The literature also includes reports of families experiencing sleep deprivation because of noisy equipment and anxiety relating to the child's condition.

With the technology often comes the need to have registered nurses or carers visiting frequently or even living with them in many cases. This is the fourth challenge. Families with a child dependent on technology are likely to share their lives with nurses and carers who can be in their homes up to 24 hours a day. This means a loss of privacy (Kirk 2005, Darvill 2003) and increases the potential for conflict.

The literature describes the importance of maintaining professional boundaries to protect family privacy and confidentiality (Hewitt-Taylor 2005, O'Brien 2001, Murphy 2001, Coffman 1995). Darvill (2003) found that the failure to maintain professional boundaries led to staff job losses, emotional problems and conflict. This study demonstrated the importance of good parental relationships and the support parents received from extended family members. These factors influenced the stability of the family unit and it was the more stable family unit that established and maintained boundaries most effectively.

Establishing good working relationships with the families

The increasingly common phenomenon of in-home care has highlighted the complexity of the family unit and the importance for nurses to be acutely aware of the significance and intricacy of a working relationship in a family home. The partnerships that form with families are important (Kirk 2005, Henry 2004, Lindeke et al. 2002, Dixon 1996, Diehl et al. 1991). The use of a tool such as the family management styles framework (Deatrick et al. 2006) may assist nurses to identify family management styles and subsequent support needs.

Over time, families develop expertise in caring for the child who is technology dependent and the parents' body of knowledge may eventually equate or surpass that of the nurse and consequently blur the usual boundaries between the 'non-expert' layperson and the 'expert' health professional (Kirk & Glendinning 2002). Regardless of the parents' expertise, parents must have ongoing access to nursing advice, reassurance and information. Ideally, this support should be available 24 hours a day.

Nurses working in community settings need to negotiate good working relationships with families so that there is mutual recognition of knowledge and expertise. Failure to do so can lead to anger and distress for the parents and potential harm for the child (Kirk & Glendinning 2002). To establish and maintain good working relationships, nurses need to not only have proficient knowledge and clinical expertise, but also be expert communicators, negotiating and coordinating services, engaging in education with clients, and providing counselling and emotional support (Kirk & Glendinning 2002).

Conclusion

Chronic illness in children and young people differs from that in adulthood and there are areas of significant concern. The diagnosis of a chronic illness means the end of life as it was known for the child/young person, their parents and siblings. There are a wide number of issues and problems that families may encounter as they try to normalise their new situations. The transition from child to adult-based care requires unique support services that are beginning to emerge.

Children/young people who are dependent on technology are both chronically ill and reliant on a technological device. They and their families face many of the same issues and problems as the family with a chronically ill child/young person; however, the degrees of difference between these two groups have not yet been researched. Technology dependence brings unique challenges, often requiring considerably more support. This can be provided as an individualised care package. Success is dependent on the adequacy of the package and developing a culturally appropriate partnership with the family that acknowledges their skills and expertise. Also nurses require high levels of skill, particularly in communicating, counselling, educating and service coordination.

Children and young people are capable of expressing their perspective, which may differ from that of their parents. Their point of view should be taken into account in both nursing management and service planning.

Practice tips

» Identify and use tools to assess families' responses to having a chronically ill or technology-dependent child.
» Use assessment findings to advocate for / provide individualised services.
» Develop / provide for the development of high levels of communication, teaching and planning skills.
» Begin planning discharge early with the family, child / young person and relevant services.
» Listen to the perspective of the child / young person.

Useful resources

Australasian Paediatric Endocrine Group: www.racp.edu.au / apeg / .
Australian Department of Health and Ageing: www.health.gov.au / .
Australian Institute of Health and Welfare: www.aihw.gov.au / .
Children's Hospitals Australasia: www.wcha.asn.au / index.cfm / spid / 1_9.cfm.
Ministry of Health New Zealand: www.moh.govt.nz / moh.nsf.
National Asthma Council Australia: www.nationalasthma.org.au / html / home / index.asp.
New Zealand primary health care strategy: www.moh.govt.nz / primaryhealthcare.
Transition Care (New South Wales Health): www.health.nsw.gov.au / gmct / transition / resources_clinicians.html.

References

Adolescent Health Research Group 2003 *New Zealand youth: a profile of their health and well being—early findings of Youth 2000*. Available at www.youth2000.ac.nz / earlyfindings.html. Accessed 12 November 2006.

Adolescent Health Research Group 2004 *Alcohol and New Zealand youth: a snapshot of young people's experiences with alcohol*. Available at www.youth2000.ac.nz / other-reports.html. Accessed 12 November 2006.

Ambler G, Fairchild J, Craig M, Cameron F 2006 Contemporary Australian outcomes in childhood and adolescent type 1 diabetes: 10 years post the diabetes control and complications trial. *Journal of Paediatrics and Child Health* 42:403–10.

Asher MI, Barry D, Clayton T 2001 The burden of symptoms of asthma, allergic rhinoconjunctivities and atopic eczema in children and adolescents in six New Zealand centres: ISAAC phase one. *New Zealand Medical Journal* 114(1128):114–20.

Asher MI, Byrnes C (eds) 2006 *Trying to catch our breath: the burden of preventable breathing diseases in children and young people*. Asthma and Respiratory Foundation of New Zealand, Wellington. Available at www.asthmanz.co.nz/burden_of_asthma_in_nz.php.

Australian Capital Territory Government 2004 *The children's plan*. Available at www.children.act.gov.au. Accessed 19 August 2006.

Australian Institute of Health and Welfare (AIHW) 2005a *A picture of Australia's children*. Cat. No. PHE58. AIHW, Canberra.

Australian Institute of Health and Welfare (AIHW) 2005b *Selected chronic diseases among Australia's children*. Bulletin No. 29. Cat. No. AUS62. AIHW, Canberra.

Australian Institute of Health and Welfare (AIHW) 2006a *Chronic diseases and associated risk factors*. Available at www.aihw.gov.au/cdarf/index.cfm. Accessed 4 July 2006.

Australian Institute of Health and Welfare (AIHW) 2006b *Australia's health 2006: the tenth biennial health report of the Australian Institute of Health and Welfare*. Cat. No. AUS73. AIHW, Canberra.

Australian Paediatric Endocrine Group (APEG) 2005 *Clinical practice guidelines: type 1 diabetes in children and adolescents*. NHMRC, Canberra.

Baker N 2003 *Carer support needs for children and young people. A report on gaps in services for children and youth*. Child and Youth Advocacy and Expert Reference Group, Nelson, New Zealand.

Barlow JH, Ellard DR 2006 The psychosocial well-being of children with chronic disease, their parents and siblings: an overview of the research evidence base. *Child: Care, Health and Development* 32(1):19–31.

Baur L 2006 Identifying and managing childhood obesity: we can do it better. Editorial comment. *Journal of Paediatrics and Child Health* 41:401–2.

Bennett DL, Towns SJ, Steinbeck KS 2005 Smoothing the transition to adult care. *Medical Journal of Australia* 182(8):373–4.

Boosfeld B, O'Toole M 2000 Discharge planning. *Paediatric Nursing* 12(6):20–2.

Campbell-Stokes PL, Taylor BJ 2005 Prospective incidence study of diabetes mellitus in New Zealand children aged 0–14 years. *Diabetologia* 48:643–8.

Chesla CA, Rungreangkulkiji S 2001 Nursing research on family processes in chronic illness in ethnically diverse families: a decade review. *Journal of Family Nursing* 7(3):230–43.

Children's Hospitals Australasia 2005 *Clinical forum: care of children with chronic and complex healthcare needs report*. Children's Hospitals Australasia, Canberra.

Clements PT, Darvill J, Redshaw L 2006 Little voices with big messages. *Neonatal, Paediatric and Child Health Nursing* 9(3):40–6.

Coffman S 1995 Crossing lines: parents' experiences with pediatric nurses in the home. *Rehabilitation Nursing Research* 4(4):136–43.

Darvill J 2003 Families caring for children with complex health care needs at home. Thesis. Flinders University, Adelaide.

Deatrick JA, Knafl KA, Murphy-Moore C 1999 Clarifying the concept of normalization. *Image: The Journal of Nursing Scholarship* 31(3):209–13.

Deatrick JA, Thibodeaux AG, Mooney K et al. 2006 Family management style framework: a new tool with potential to assess families who have children with brain tumors. *Journal of Pediatric Oncology Nursing* 23(1):19–27.

Dellve L, Samuelsson L, Tallborn A et al. 2006 Stress and wellbeing among parents of children with rare diseases: a prospective intervention study. *Journal of Advanced Nursing* 53(4):392–402.

Department of Health 2004 *National service framework for children, young people and maternity services*. Her Majesty's Stationery Office, London.

Diehl S, Moffitt K, Wade S 1991 Focus group interview with parents of children with medically complex needs: an intimate look at their perceptions and feelings. *Children's Health Care* 20(3):170–8.

Dixon D 1996 Unifying concepts in parents' experiences with health care providers. *Journal of Family Nursing* 2:111–32.

Donaghue KC, Craig ME, Chan AKF et al. 2005 Prevalence of diabetes complications 6 years after diagnosis in an incident cohort of childhood diabetes. *Diabetic Medicine* 22:711–18.

Durie M 1994 *Whaiora. Maori health development*. Oxford University Press, Auckland.

Earle RJ, Rennick JE, Carnevale FA, Davis GM 2006 'It's okay, it helps me to breathe': the experience of home ventilation from a child's perspective. *Journal of Child Health Care* 10(4):270–82.

Edwards EA, Asher MI, Byrnes CA 2003 Paediatric bronchiectasis in the twenty-first century: experience of a tertiary children's hospital in New Zealand. *Journal of Paediatrics and Child Health* 39:111–17.

Fisher HR 2001 The needs of parents with chronically sick children: a literature review. *Journal of Advanced Nursing* 36(4):600–7.

Gilgoff RL, Gilgoff IS 2003 Long-term follow-up of home mechanical ventilation in young children with spinal cord injury and neuromuscular conditions. *Journal of Pediatrics* 142:476–80.

Glendinning C, Kirk S, Guiffrida A, Lawton D 2001 Technology dependent children in the community: definitions, numbers and costs. *Child: Care, Health and Development* 27(4):321–34.

Heaton J, Noyes J, Sloper P, Shah R 2005 Families' experiences of caring for technology dependent children: a temporal perspective. *Health and Social Care in the Community* 13(5):441–50.

Henry P 2004 Negotiating an unstable ladder: the experience of Maori families caring for a technology dependent child. Thesis. University of Auckland.

Hentinen M, Kyngas H 1998 Factors associated with the adaptation of parents with a chronically ill child. *Journal of Clinical Nursing* 7:316–24.

Hewitt-Taylor J 2005 Caring for children with complex needs: staff education and training. *Journal of Child Health Care* 9(1):72–86.

Holt M 2005 *Young people and illicit drug use in Australia*. Social Research: Issues Paper No. 3. National Centre for HIV Social Research, Sydney.

Horsburgh M, Trenholme A 2002 Respite and palliative care needs of families caring for a terminally ill child: a New Zealand study. University of Auckland.

Jardine E, Wallis C 1998 Core guidelines for the discharge home of the child on long term assisted ventilation in the United Kingdom. *Thorax* 53:762–7.

Kirk S 1998 Families' experiences of caring at home for a technology dependent child: a review of the literature. *Child: Care, Health and Development* 24(2):101–14.

Kirk S 2005 Parent or nurse? The experience of being the parent of a technology-dependent child. *Journal of Advanced Nursing* 51(5):456–64.

Kirk S, Glendinning C 2002 Supporting 'expert' parents: professional support and families caring for a child with complex health care needs in the community. *International Journal of Nursing Studies* 39:625–35.

Knafl K, Breitmayer B, Gallo A, Zoeller L 1996 Family response to childhood chronic illness: description of management styles. *Journal of Pediatric Nursing* 11(5):315–26.

Knafl K, Deatrick JA 2002 The challenge of normalization for families of children with chronic conditions. *Pediatric Nursing* 28(1):49–53.

Knafl K, Deatrick JA 2006 Family management style and the challenge of moving from conceptualization to measurement. *Journal of Pediatric Oncology Nursing* 23(1):12–18.

Krulik T, Turner-Henson A, Kanematsu Y et al. 1999 Parenting stress and mothers of young children with chronic illness: a cross cultural study. *Journal of Pediatric Nursing* 14(2):130–40.

Kyngas H 2000 Compliance of adolescents with chronic disease. *Journal of Clinical Nursing* 9:549–56.

Kyngas H, Rissanen M 2001 Support as a crucial predictor of good compliance of adolescents with a chronic disease. *Journal of Clinical Nursing* 10(6):767–73.

Lean M, Lara J, O'Hill J 2006 Strategies for preventing obesity. *British Medical Journal* 333:959–62.

Lindeke L, Leonard B, Presler B, Garwick A 2002 Family-centered care coordination for children with special needs across multiple settings. *Journal of Pediatric Health Care* 16(6):290–7.

Melnyk BM, Feinstein NF, Moldenhouer Z, Small L 2001 Coping in parents of children who are chronically ill: strategies for assessment and intervention. *Pediatric Nursing* 27(6):548–58, 572–3.

Mentro A, Steward D 2002 Caring for medically fragile children in the home: an alternative theoretical approach. *Research and Theory for Nursing Practice* 16(3):161–77.

Miller S 2002 Respite care for children who have complex healthcare needs. *Paediatric Nursing* 14(5):33–7.

Ministry of Health New Zealand (MOH NZ) 1998 *Our children's health*. MOH NZ, Wellington.

Ministry of Health New Zealand (MOH NZ) 2004 *Statistics New Zealand*. Available at www.stats.govt.nz/analytical-reports/children-in-nz/disability.htm.

Ministry of Health New Zealand (MOH NZ) 2006 *An analysis of the usefulness and feasibility of a population indicator of childhood obesity*. MOH NZ, Wellington.

Murphy G 2001 The technology-dependent child at home part 1: in whose best interest? *Paediatric Nursing* 13(7):14–18.

National Asthma Council Australia (NAC) 2006 *Asthma management handbook 2006*. NAC, Melbourne.

Neufeld S, Query B, Drummond J 2001 Respite care users who have children with chronic conditions: are they getting a break? *Journal of Pediatric Nursing* 16(4):234–44.

Noyes J 2000 Enabling young ventilator dependent people to express their views and experiences of their care in hospital. *Journal of Advanced Nursing* 31(5):1206–15.

Noyes J 2002 Barriers that delay children and young people who are dependent on mechanical ventilators from being discharged from hospital. *Journal of Clinical Nursing* 11:2–11.

Noyes J 2006a Health and quality of life of ventilator-dependent children. *Journal of Advanced Nursing* 56(4):392–403.

Noyes J 2006b The key to success: managing children's complex packages of community support. *Archives of Diseases in Childhood. Education and Practice* 91:106–10. doi:10.1136/adc.2005.088351.

Noyes J 2007 Comparison of ventilator-dependent child reports of health-related quality of life with parent reports and normative populations. *Journal of Advanced Nursing* 58(1):1–10.

O'Brien M 2001 Living in a house of cards: family experiences with long term childhood technology dependence. *Journal of Pediatric Nursing* 16(1):13–22.

O'Halloran J, Miller G, Britt H 2004 Defining chronic conditions for primary care for ICPC-2. *Family Practice* 21(4):381–6.

Santrock J 2004 *Child development*, 10th edn. McGraw Hill, New York.

Sartain SA, Clarke CL, Heyman R 2000 Hearing the voices of children with chronic illness. *Journal of Advanced Nursing* 32(4):913–21.

Stein REK 2001 Challenges in long term healthcare for children. *Ambulatory Pediatrics* 1(5):280–8.

Steinbeck K, Brodie L 2006 Bringing in the voices: a transition forum for young people with chronic illness or disability. *Neonatal, Paediatric and Child Health Nursing* 9(1):22–6.

United Nations (UN) 1989 *Convention on the rights of the child*. Available at www.ohchr.org/english/law/pdf/crc.pdf. Accessed 17 December 2006.

Woodgate R 2001 Adopting the qualitative paradigm to understanding children's perspectives of illness: barrier or facilitator. *Journal of Pediatric Nursing* 16(3):149–61.

Index

Page numbers followed by 'f' denote figures, 't' denote tables, and 'b' denote boxes.

O

P